Manual of

Postpartum Hemorrhage and High-Risk Pregnancy

Manual of
Postpartum Hemorrhage and High-Risk Pregnancy

Editors

SN Tripathy

KC Mahapatra

SK Giri

Sheela Mane

Palaniappan

Sasmita Swain

61st AICOG 2018 Odisha

61st AICOG BHUBANESWAR 2018

JAYPEE *The Health Sciences Publisher*

New Delhi | London | Panama

Jaypee Brothers Medical Publishers (P) Ltd

Headquarters
Jaypee Brothers Medical Publishers (P) Ltd
4838/24, Ansari Road, Daryaganj
New Delhi 110 002, India
Phone: +91-11-43574357
Fax: +91-11-43574314
Email: jaypee@jaypeebrothers.com

Overseas Offices

J.P. Medical Ltd
83 Victoria Street, London
SW1H 0HW (UK)
Phone: +44-20 317 08910
Fax: +44 (0)20 3008 6180
Email: info@jpmedpub.com

Jaypee-Highlights Medical Publishers Inc
City of Knowledge, Bld. 235, 2nd floor, Clayton
Panama City, Panama
Phone: +1 507-301-0496
Fax: +1 507-301-0499
Email: cservice@jphmedical.com

Jaypee Brothers Medical Publishers (P) Ltd
17/1-B Babar Road, Block-B, Shyamoli
Mohammadpur, Dhaka-1207
Bangladesh
Mobile: +08801912003485
Email: jaypeedhaka@gmail.com

Jaypee Brothers Medical Publishers (P) Ltd
Bhotahity, Kathmandu, Nepal
Phone: +977-9741283608
Email: Kathmandu@jaypeebrothers.com

Website: www.jaypeebrothers.com
Website: www.jaypeedigital.com

Inquiries for bulk sales may be solicited at: jaypee@jaypeebrothers.com

Manual of Postpartum Hemorrhage and High-Risk Pregnancy

First Edition: **2018**

ISBN 978-93-5270-370-8

Printed at

Contributors

Chaitali Dutta
Associate Professor
Department of Obstetrics and Gynecology
Kolkata, West Bengal, India

Gangadhar Sahoo
Dean
Department of Obstetrics and Gynecology
Sambalpur, Odisha, India

Joydev Mukherjee
Professor
Department of Obstetrics and Gynecology
Kolkata, West Bengal, India

Leena Das
Department of Obstetrics and Gynecology
Bhubaneswar, Odisha, India

Lucy Das
Professor
Department of Obstetrics and Gynecology
Cuttack, Odisha, India

Mamta Rath Datta
Head Consultant
Department of Obstetrics and Gynecology
Jamshedpur, Jharkhand, India

Samartha Ram
Director, and Senior Consultant
Department of Obstetrics and Gynecology
Palakkad, Kerala, India

Sheela V Mane
Consultant
Department of Obstetrics and Gynecology
Bengaluru, Karnataka, India

Smita Mahapatra
Associate Professor
Cuttack, Odisha, India

SN Routray
Professor and Head
Department of Cardiology
Cuttack, Odisha, India

Sujata Misra
Associate Professor
Cuttack, Odisha, India

Sukumar Barik
Department of Obstetrics and Gynecology
Kolkata, West Bengal, India

Tushar Kar
Professor and Head
Department of Obstetrics and Gynecology
Veer Surendra Sai Institute of Medical Sciences and Research (VIMSAR)
Sambalpur, Odisha, India

Message

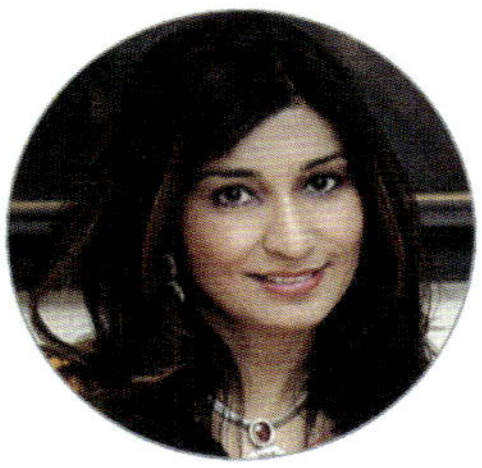

Rishma Dhillon Pai
MD DNB FCPS DGO FICOG
President, FOGSI—2017
Consultant Gynecologist
Jaslok Hospital, Lilavati Hospital and Hinduja Healthcare (Khar),
Bloom IVF Centre,
The Every Woman Clinic,
Mumbai, Maharashtra, India

"Wisdom.... comes not from age, but from education and learning."
Anton Chekhov

Life is a continuous process of learning. Especially in the field of medicine, which is constantly changing, it is very important to keep oneself abreast with the latest developments. It is heartening to note that academic workshop manuals are being released at the AICOG, Bhubaneswar, Odisha, India, for the benefit of the participating delegates and present varied updates in the field. Many different Manuals are being released on important subjects such as *3D Laparoscopy and Operative Oncology, Genetics, Fetal Medicine and Color Doppler, Postpartum Hemorrhage and High-Risk Pregnancy, Hysteroscopy,* etc.

I thank all the authors, for their immense contributions in building up the content for the manuals for Federation of Obstetric and Gynaecological Societies of India (FOGSI) by sharing their rich experiences in the field. These will be a big help to young gynecologists, who are still acquiring skills in various aspects of obstetrics and gynecology and a quick update for the seniors.

I extend congratulations to the organizing team of the AICOG 2018 and the editors of these manuals and wish you all success for this mega event.

"You cannot open a book without learning something."

—Confucius

Message

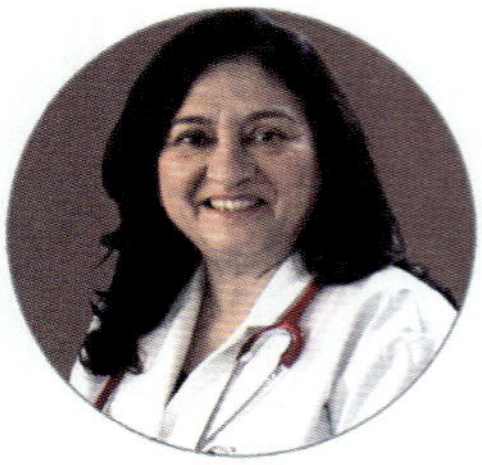

Jaideep Malhotra
MD FICMCH FICS FMAS FRCOG FICOG FRCPI FIAJAGO
Consultant ART (IVF)
President Elect, FOGSI—2018
Director, Rainbow IVF
Agra, Uttar Pradesh, India

"Education is greatest gift of life, it should never stop."

The subject of obstetrics and gynecology needs extreme proficiency as it deals with the medical specialties that focus on two different aspects. First one includes the care of pregnant women, the unborn baby, labor and delivery, as well as the immediate period following childbirth. Second aspect includes dealing with any ailment concerning the female reproductive organs. Hence, the manuals will help all those who are looking forward to gain excellence in the field of woman health. The manuals have tried to address all the issues a doctor needs.

With increasing expertise in all fields, the surgeon therefore while exercising a choice needs to follow the Hippocratic dictum—*"First, do no harm."*

We are thankful to all those who have incorporated their contribution by providing chapters from their research and collected scientific material and have shared their fruitful experiences for the delegates of the workshop.

As a part of my agenda for 2018, I as FOGSI President 2018, plan to work actively on QED (Quality, Ethics and Dignity) among our profession and also work towards HER (Health, Empowerment and Respect) towards our patients.

"Knowledge is of no value unless you put it into practices."

Message

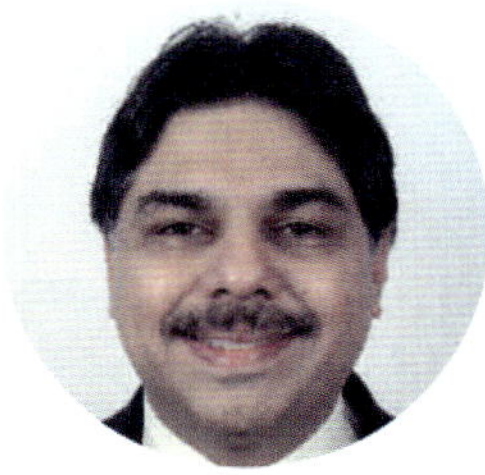

Hrishikesh Pai
Secretary General, FOGSI

It is my proud privilege to invite and welcome all delegates to the 61st All India Congress of Obstetrics and Gynaecology (AICOG) from 17th–21st January, 2018 at the Temple City of India, Bhubaneswar, Odisha, India.

It is propitious to note that the academic workshop manuals are being released which will reap beneficial reward to all the participating delegates.

I thank all the authors, for their immense contributions in building up the content for the manuals for Federation of Obstetric and Gynaecological Societies of India (FOGSI) by sharing their rich experiences in the field. These will be a big help to young gynecologists, who are still acquiring skills in various aspects of obstetrics and gynecology and a quick update for the seniors.

I forward my heartiest congratulations to all the contributors, the editors and the delegates of the workshop.

Message

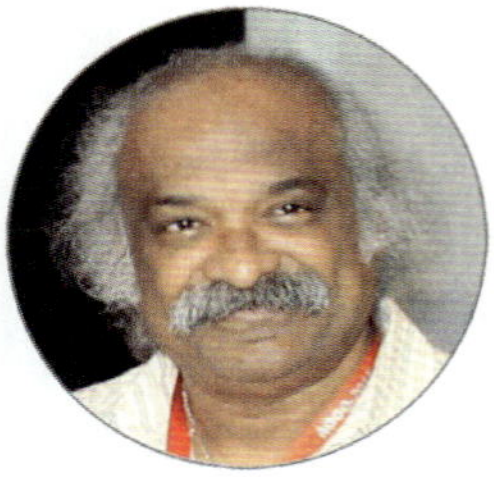

PC Mahapatra
Professor
Department of Obstetrics and Gynecology
SCB Medical College
Cuttack, Odisha, India
President, FOGSI—2011
Organising Chairperson

It is my proud privilege to invite and welcome all delegates to the 61st All India Congress of Obstetrics and Gynaecology (AICOG) from 17th–21st January, 2018 at the Temple City of India, Bhubaneswar, Odisha, India.

The five days of academic extravaganza will certainly enrich the scientific knowledge of all participating delegates and faculty. The precongress workshop on various aspects of this specialty will be held on 17th January 2018.

A quote by Edwin Louis Cole says that "*Winners are not those who never fail but those who never quit*" is apt for all the clinicians who are determined enough to see and overcome all the difficulties that are faced in the field of obstetrics and gynecology.

Today, with the advancement in the field of obstetrics and gynecology, everyone requires an in-depth knowledge of the complex subjects associated with the field so as to gain excellence in it.

This manual will prove to be a boon to all those who are associated with the field and wants to gain more knowledge in the subject matter.

Message

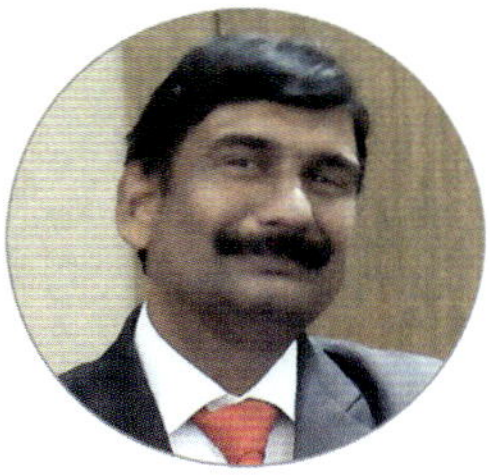

HP Pattanaik
Head
Department of Obstetrics and Gynecology
City Hospital
Cuttack, Odisha, India
Vice President, FOGSI—2009
Organising Secretary

Greetings from 61st AICOG 2018!
It is a matter of great pleasure to invite you all to 61st AICOG, from 17th–21st January, 2018 at the Temple City of India, Bhubaneswar, Odisha, India. The 11th Precongress workshops will be held on 17th January, 2018 in three medical colleges of Bhubaneswar.

It is propitious to note that the academic workshop manuals are being released which will reap beneficial reward to all the participating delegates.

It will also prove to be beneficial to the members of Federation of Obstetric and Gynaecological Societies of India (FOGSI), those who were unable to register themselves for the academic workshops.

I forward my heartiest congratulations to all the contributors, the editors and the delegates of the workshop.

Preface

The basic fact of today is the tremendous pace of change in human life.

Jawaharlal Nehru.

So also science is progressing in leaps and bounds. Still we are not able to predict postpartum hemorrhage (PPH). It is not very clear why some women develop atonic PPH and why some women do not? PPH affects approximately 2% of all women who give birth and is associated with nearly one quarter of all maternal deaths globally. The reported incidence of PPH in India is 2%–4% after vaginal delivery and 6% after cesarean section with uterine atony being the most common cause (50%).

The only management strategy even today is 'watchful expectancy' and act immediately when the problem arises. Simpler techniques like uterine massage, uterotonic drugs, and uterine packing and balloon tamponade can be practiced in low resource settings. Techniques like B-Lynch suturing, stepwise devascularization, internal iliac ligation and uterine artery embolization are available only at higher medical centers. These higher techniques are not within the reach of every parturient woman when simpler techniques fail. In low resource settings, unpredictable sudden massive bleeding makes it difficult to organize competent manpower, compatible blood and transport to higher medical center. Many times mothers die on roads while being transported to higher medical centers due to hypovolemic shock. Sometimes, women succumb to death just within 1–1.5 hours after the onset of bleeding. There is every need for a simpler and sure technique which can stop bleeding, or at least stop bleeding temporarily to buy some time to tide over the crisis.

To be frank, there is no high-risk group, but all pregnancies are at risk. Amongst them, there is a group who require a little more attention. Cardiovascular disease (CVD) affects 0.2–4% of pregnant women but account for one-third of all pregnancy-related deaths. The maternal mortality in CVD patients is about 1% which is 100 times more than the normal pregnant population. While modern medicine enables an increasing number of CHD patients to attain childbearing age, ischemic heart disease incidence is also rising due to advancing maternal age and risk factors (smoking, obesity, diabetes and hypertension. The magnitude of the problem is so great that it demand is the attention of all health care personnel involved in maternal and child care. Membrane rupture before labor and before 37 weeks of gestation is referred to as preterm prematrue rupture of membranes (PROM). Preterm prematrue rupture of membranes (PPROM) is far more difficult to manage than premature rupture of membranes at term. The condition increases fetal mortality and maternal morbidity. The management of PPROM depends on the balance between the risks for fetal and neonatal complications with immediate delivery versus the risks and benefits of conservative treatment.

Jaundice in pregnancy has many etiologies. The condition must be properly evaluated. Proper management may improve maternal and fetal outcome. Twin pregnancy always poses problems, The problem anticipated and should be managed properly. As obstetrician are the first person to receive a baby during delivery, all of them should be trained in the art of neonatal resuscitation. Many such topics are included in the workshop and stalwarts in the field will enlighten us about the subjects. Listening, participating in a close group enhances our knowledge to a great extent. Knowledge is the key to success and our success means caring for the suffering diseased women in a better way. Happy reading.

Editors

Content

1. **Postpartum Hemorrhage—The Present Scenario, How Far We have Succeeded and Way Forward** 1
Gangadhar Sahoo

2. **Traumatic Postpartum Hemorrhage—The Forgotten Entity** 5
Tushar Kar

3. **Medical Management of Postpartum Hemorrhage: The Present Guidelines** 7
Joydev Mukherji

4. **Massive Transfusion Protocol—What, How, and How Much?** 12
Smita Mahapatra

5. **Nonpneumatic Antishock Garment** 15
Gomathy Narayanan

6. **Uterine Tamponade: The Newer Methods, Controversies and Consensus** 21
H Samartha Ram

7. **Management of Postpartum Hemorrhage: Where Do We Go Wrong?** 27
Sabaratnam Arulkumaran

8. **Heart Disease in Pregnancy: A Cardiologist Message to Obstetricians** 29
SN Routray

9. **Jaundice in Pregnancy—Maternal and Fetal Outcome** 34
Mamta Rath Datta

10. **Management of Monochorionic Twins** 42
Lucy Das

11. **Unexplained Fetal Death** 49
Chaitali Dutta

12. **Preterm Premature Rupture of Membranes—An Enigma** 54
Sukumar Barik

13. **Screening and Management of Gestational Diabetes** 58
Sujata Misra

14. **Neonatal Resuscitation: A Skill Every Obstetrician Should Know** 66
Leena Das

Chapter 1

Postpartum Hemorrhage—The Present Scenario, How Far We have Succeeded and Way Forward

Gangadhar Sahoo

POSTPARTUM HEMORRHAGE—THE PRESENT SCENARIO

The vast disparities between regions and countries in maternal health have long been known. The most recent estimates show that in 2008, maternal mortality ratios (MMRs) ranged from 290 maternal deaths per 100,000 live births in developing countries to just 14 in developed countries. The fact that an estimated 385,000 women die each year during pregnancy, delivery, and the postpartum period suggests inadequate overall progress toward reproductive health, including maternal health. Furthermore, there is a growing body of evidence showing that even within countries; maternal health outcomes are inequitably distributed, with the poorest likely to be most disadvantaged.

GLOBAL BURDEN OF POSTPARTUM HEMORRHAGE

Postpartum hemorrhage (PPH) affects approximately 2% of all women who give birth and is associated with nearly one quarter of all maternal deaths globally. The exact rates may differ according to data source, country as well as assessment method with prevalence of 10.6% when measured by objective assessment of blood loss and 7.2% when measured by subjective techniques. Prevalence of PPH more than or equal to 500 mL ranged from 2.55% in Asia to 10.45% in Africa. PPH accounts for 25% of maternal mortality in Africa. Half of all the maternal deaths worldwide occur in Africa. These deaths have been a direct result of the defects in the social, cultural, and economic status of women as well as inadequacies in existing health systems. In 2010, approximately 280,000 women died due to complications of pregnancy and childbirth; 995 of these deaths occur in developing countries and almost all could have been prevented. The reported incidence of PPH in India is 2–4% after vaginal delivery and 6% after cesarean section with uterine atony being the most common cause (50%). WHO estimates that of the 5,29,000 maternal death occurring every year, 1,36,000 or 25.7% of death takes place in India and two-thirds of these maternal death occur after delivery.

POSTPARTUM HEMORRHAGE AND THE MILLENNIUM DEVELOPMENT GOALS

One of the targets of the Millennium Development Goal 5 was to reduce the MMR by three quarters between 1990 and 2015. In the developing regions as a whole the MMR dropped by 34% between 1990 and 2008 (from 440 to 290 maternal deaths per 100,000 live births). The Millennium Development Goal target, however, is still far off. The MMR in India between 2007 and 2009 was 212, which is far away from the Millennium Development Goal 5 target for India: 109 maternal deaths per 100,000 live births.

HOW FAR WE HAVE SUCCEEDED?

Postpartum hemorrhage is a frequent complication of delivery and its reported incidence in India is 2–4% after vaginal delivery and 6% after cesarean section with uterine atony being the most common cause (50%). Furthermore latest figures report PPH as the contributory cause of 19.9% of maternal mortality, that is anywhere from 78,000 to 117,000 maternal deaths in India. With 56,000 maternal deaths, India accounted for 19% of global burden of maternal deaths in 2010, though it has only 16% of global population. The level of MMR in India has declined from 254 in 2004–2006 to 212 in 2007–2009, but it has not yet reached the desired levels. The prevention and treatment of PPH are vital steps toward improving the healthcare of women during childbirth and the achievement of the Millennium Development Goals. The current scenario in developing countries mandates research on newer and practicable strategies to tackle PPH which can be implemented effectively and have an upper edge over the existing practices in the management of PPH. Our approach to emergency obstetric care crawls at Snail's Pace.

PREVENTION

Most deaths resulting from PPH occur during the first 24 hours after birth. Appropriate management of women during the third stage of labor will prevent the majority of these deaths. Active management of the third stage of labor (AMTSL) lowers maternal blood loss and reduces the risk of PPH (Cochrane reviews of 2000 and 2011). As the majority of women who experience PPH complications have no identifiable clinical or historical risk factors, it is recommended that AMTSL be offered to all women during childbirth, whenever a skilled provider is assisting with the delivery.

CHALLENGES IN PREVENTION OF MATERNAL MORTALITY IN POSTPARTUM HEMORRHAGE

Research by the Prevention of Maternal Mortality Project has drawn the importance of essential obstetrics care (EOC), particularly emergency care in reducing maternal mortality. Three factors of delay contribute to mortality:
1. The decision to seek EOC
2. Delay in transportation
3. Delay in obtaining treatment once the patient is in the facility.

The active management of third stage of labor is a well-established evidence-based intervention for the prevention of uterine atony—the most common cause of PPH—but it is not widely used in some developing countries. In the year 2007, WHO developed a set of guidelines for the prevention of PPH which highlights the importance of the active management. But healthcare systems face enormous challenges due to financial constraint that affect the delivery of EOC. Moreover many deliveries are still performed by untrained persons, especially in rural areas and this fact leads to a greater degree of nonrecognition of the dangers of PPH.

WAYS TO PREVENT PPH

One of the ways to prevent PPH is AMTSL. It is considered to be the "gold standard" to reduce the incidence of PPH. Studies have compared AMTSL with expectant management and found a substantial reduction in the occurrence of PPH by approximately 60–70%. Furthermore, the most recent Cochrane review of active versus expectant management of third stage of labor including seven studies indicates a significant reduction in risk of PPH with AMTSL. In my opinion along with improvement of application of obstetric knowledge and skill our main objectives should be control and stabilization of population, change in lifestyle of young women, rendering health education, and providing skilled service at the primary care level.

A LONG WAY FORWARD

Resources, power, and access to opportunities are unequally and unfairly distributed across social categories, creating social gradients that disadvantage people in lower social positions. Relationships with male partners are another factor that affects women's health. The level of a husband's education is also a major determinant of skilled attendance at birth, indicating that women might need to take husband's or partner's permission before taking decisions related to care.

Additional research is needed to determine the most effective treatments of PPH. Clinicians should follow consensus guidelines, expert opinions, and local protocols to manage PPH. It is important for clinicians to recognize PPH as it occurs and not to delay instituting guideline-based measures to control bleeding. Hence, a lot needs to be done at individual, community, and political levels to promote maternal health and to reduce the burden of maternal deaths in India. Prevention of maternal deaths in resource-poor countries remains a challenge. But, implementation of interventions to achieve the Millennium Goals may be a confident way forward.

PPH was there, PPH is here, and PPH will remain in future. It is very difficult to predict if the severity of this catastrophe will change.

I foresee the incidence of PPH will rise in future due to:

- Dying interest in obstetric practice by the physicians
- Change in lifestyle of women in reproductive age group who are opting for assisted reproductive technique (ART) and cesarean section.
- Callousness and apathy at the social and political level.

Mothers are destined to bleed, they bleed for a noble cause. But they should not bleed to death or develop a morbidity during child birth in modern obstetric practice.

In the present scenario, I feel it is too difficult to dispel the apprehension of the Tanzanian mother "Mother I am going to deep sea to fetch a baby. I do not know if I can return."

Pray God to bail the obstetricians out of this terrible but preventable catastrophe. Only He can save.

Chapter 2

Traumatic Postpartum Hemorrhage—The Forgotten Entity

Tushar Kar

"Taj Mahal—a tear drop on the check of time" was created in the memory of Mumtaz Mahal who died of postpartum hemorrhage (PPH) during her fourteenth confinement in 1631. Centuries have passed, but PPH remains a leading cause of maternal morbidity and mortality and accounts for a one-fourth to half of maternal deaths worldwide.

Population-based surveys have reported a wide variation in the prevalence of PPH form 5% to 17.5%. The challenge is that the reduction in mortality cannot be achieved just by enhancing skills and technology but will require strategies.

The various causes of PPH are atonic, traumatic, retained placental bits, coagulation disorder, mixed variety and placenta accreta. Traumatic PPH contributes to 10–20% of all PPH. Various types of trauma may be laceration of cervix, vagina and perineum (vulvar hematoma) and paraurethral tear. Others may be due to rupture of uterus, extension of cesarean section (CS) wound, broad ligament hematoma and uterine inversion. Predisposing factors for traumatic PPH may be delivery through undilated cervix like precipitate labor or by excessive fundal pressure. Others may be due to instrumental delivery or face to pubis delivery.

Out of all traumas vulvar hematoma may be forgotten at times. Proper perineal examination can detect vulvar hematoma. The lower genital trauma can be anterior vaginal tears with/without urethral or clitoral involvement, lateral vaginal wall tears, posterior vaginal tears, invariably involving anal triangle of perineum, spiral vaginal tears, colporrhexis, vulval injuries and episiotomies. Posteriorly vaginal or perineal tears may be first, second, third and fourth degree. First degree is injury to perineal skin only. Second degree is injury to perineum involving perineal muscles but not involving anal sphincters. Third degree tear is injury to perineum involving the anal sphincter complex. Third degree A is less than 50% of external anal sphincter torn, 3B is more than 50% of anal sphincter torn, and 3C: both external and internal anal sphincter torn. Fourth degree is injury to perineum involving the anal sphincter complex and anal epithelium. Perineal tears can be associated with significant morbidity and to lesser extent even mortality. The primary aim of an obstetrician is to reduce the incidence of these injuries, followed by correct recognition and management.

Cervical tears can lead to brisk blood loss. Exploration of cervix and repair of lateral tears should be done immediately following vaginal delivery in traumatic PPH. Cervical laceration at cesarean delivery may be difficult to repair and may require hysterectomy. Presence of cervical cerclage and bearing down prior to complete cervical dilation are risk factors for cervical tears. Infralevator hematomas are common and easily diagnosed on vulval inspection. They may be managed conservatively or require surgical drainage. Supralevator hematomas are uncommon and may lead to hemodynamic instability. They are diagnosed by USG or CT/MRI for complete mapping. They are managed by either laparotomy or transfemoral selective arterial embolization. Hematomas can be prevented by meticulous attention to hemostasis.

Morbidly adherent placenta is associated with a high maternal mortality. Careful sonological assessment of uteroplacental interface is required in patients with previous uterine scars and placenta previa. Surgical management consists of classical CS without disturbing placental site. Further management may be an obstetric hysterectomy or a conservative approach of leaving the placenta in situ and administering methotrexate under broad spectrum antibiotic cover. Uterine artery embolization is done after delivery of fetus to minimize blood loss. Massive transfusion of blood and blood products may be required.

Rupture of uterus is an immediate emergency with high maternal morbidity and mortality necessitating immediate resuscitation and laparotomy. Uterine rupture may be of complete or incomplete types. Etiologically, the rupture may be spontaneous, due to scar rupture, instrumental delivery or at times iatrogenic. Spontaneous rupture in labor may be due to obstruction, grand multi or due to oxytocic and prostaglandin use. For scar dehiscence, repair can be tried. Most rupture have irregular ragged margin and usually need subtotal or total hysterectomy.

Inversion of uterus is extremely rare but a life-threatening complication of 3rd stage. This may be 1st degree, 2nd degree and 3rd degree. It may be acute, subacute or chronic. In 1st degree, fundus is depressed up to internal os, in 2nd degree the fundus comes out through external us into the vagina but not outside vagina. In 3rd degree uterus and cervix are completely inverted. In acute inversion, quick manual reposition is done under general anesthesia, if it fails O'Sullivan's hydrostatic method is done to repose the uterus. Other methods of reposition of inversion uterus are Huntington technique, Haultain's technique and Spinelle's technique.

Chapter 3

Medical Management of Postpartum Hemorrhage: The Present Guidelines

Joydev Mukherji

INTRODUCTION

No single satisfactory definition of postpartum hemorrhage (PPH) exists and a number of definitions are currently in use worldwide.

NEED FOR HOSPITAL SPECIFIC PROTOCOLS

Almost all guidelines, recommend instituting a policy or establishing a protocol when PPH is identified, yet the specifics to the protocol vary.[1]

The essential elements of a system that guarantees the speed and effectiveness essential to controlling PPH are a department protocol that is regularly updated and trained staff who communicate correctly.[2.]

PPH Kits: In addition to a protocol, it is useful for labor and delivery units to assemble kits that contain medications and instruments that may be needed to manage PPH.[3]

TRANSFER TO APPROPRIATE CENTER

The ambulance transfer with medical accompaniment can be performed only after correction of any life-threatening failure.[2.]

Transfer with Ongoing Intravenous Uterotonic Infusion

Be ready at all times to transfer to a higher level facility if the patient is not responding to the treatment or a treatment cannot be administered at home/ facility. Ensure client will get assured services at higher referral centers.[4]

ESTIMATION OF PERIPARTUM BLOOD LOSS

The visual estimation of peripartum blood loss is inaccurate and that clinical signs and symptoms should be included in the assessment of PPH.[5.]

Some guidelines invoke basic measures for estimated blood loss (EBL) of 500–1,000 mL with no clinical shock and a full protocol of measures for EBL greater than 1,000 mL and continuing bleeding, or where there is evidence of clinical shock. It is important to consider both the patient's prior hemoglobin and her total blood volume when assessing the severity of PPH.[6.]

MULTIDISCIPLINARY TEAM

Team may include obstetricians, nurses, anesthesiologists, hematologists/ blood bank personnel, laboratory medicine, surgical subspecialists (e.g. urology), and interventional radiologists.[4,5]

TEMPORIZING MEASURES

World Health Organization[7]

Temporizing measures (until appropriate care is available):
- Bimanual uterine compression
- External aortic compression
- Non-pneumatic antishock garments.

Royal College of Obstetricians and Gynecologists[8]

Compression of the aorta may be a temporary but effective measure to allow time for resuscitation to catch up with the volume replacement and the appropriate surgical support to arrive.

Pneumatic antishock gear is a temporizing measure if available, although does not specify when, in the management schema, it should be used.[8.]

MANAGEMENT OF POSTPARTUM HEMORRHAGE

There is little randomized control trial (RCT) evidence to guide the management of PPH.[6]

First-line Therapy

The first-line therapy is usually medical management. The simple mechanical and physiological measures of "rubbing up the fundus" and emptying the bladder to stimulate uterine contraction.
- *Uterotonic agents* should be the first-line pharmacological treatment for atony.[7]

- *Oxytocin:* When given as an intravenous (IV) bolus the drug should be given slowly in a dose of not more than 5 IU.[8]
- A *second uterotonic* agent is required in 3–25% of cases of PPH.
- Supplemental uterotonics that are most commonly administered include methylergonovine, 15-methyl prostaglandin F_2 alpha, or misoprostol. There is a lack of evidence to suggest which specific additional uterotonics are the most effective.[5]
- *Misoprostol*
  - The optimum dose and route of are unclear
  - Recommended sublingually (WHO 800 µg)
  - Government of India (GOI 2015)—if bleeding is not controlled after use of oxytocin, it is recommended to switch over to the next uterotonic IV methergine, or sublingual misoprostol 800 µg.[4]

Resuscitation

[Modified from Royal College of Obstetricians and Gynaecologists (RCOG) 2016]

- Intravenous access (one 14-gauge cannula)
- Foley catheter for emptying bladder and recording urine volume
- Urgent venepuncture (20 mL) for group and screen, full blood count, coagulation screen
- Pulse, respiratory rate and BP monitoring every 15 minutes
- Commence warmed crystalloid infusion
- Maintain oxygenation
- Avoid hypothermia and acidosis.

Coagulation Abnormalities

Tranexamic Acid

The "WOMAN" trial demonstrated efficacy of 1 g of tranexamic acid IV with a clinical diagnosis of PPH.[6]

As treatment for PPH, tranexamic acid should be given as soon as possible after bleeding onset.[9]

GOI (2015)—tranexamic acid is recommended for the treatment of PPH if oxytocin and other uterotonics fail to stop the bleeding or the bleeding may be partly due to trauma.[4]

In most cases, therapy of PPH cannot be based on the actual hemostatic competence because regular conventional coagulation tests typically require 45–60 minutes for results to be available and are nonspecific.

Red blood cells (RBCs), fibrinogen and fresh frozen plasma (FFP) may be administered without awaiting laboratory results (Box 3.1).[2]

When treating PPH, it is necessary to balance the use of less invasive management techniques with the need to control the bleeding and achieve hemostasis.[5]

Box 3.1: Volume replacement: Intravenous fluids, blood and blood products

1. *Crystalloid:* Up to 2 l isotonic crystalloid
2. *Colloid:* Up to 1.5 L colloid till blood arrives
3. *Blood:* If immediate transfusion is indicated, give emergency group O, rhesus D (RhD)-negative, K-negative red cell units. Switch to group specific red cells as soon as available
4. *FFP:* Administration should be guided by hemostatic testing and whether hemorrhage is continuing:
   I. If PT or APTT are prolonged or hemorrhage is ongoing administer 12–15 mL/kg of FFP
   II. If hemorrhage continues after 4 units of red blood cells and hemostatic tests are unavailable administer 4 units of FFP
5. *Platelets:* Administer one pool of platelets if hemorrhage is ongoing and platelet count is <75 × 109
6. *Cryoprecipitate:* Administer two pools of cryoprecipitate if hemorrhage is ongoing and fibrinogen is <2 g/L
7. *Tranexamic acid*
8. *Recombinant factor VIIa (rFVIIa):* Not recommended unless part of a clinical trial

(FFP: fresh frozen plasma; APTT: activated partial thromboplastin time; PT: prothrombin time)
Source: Modified from RCOG.

MONITORING

Vital Signs

Evaluate blood pressure, heart rate, respiratory rate, peripheral oxygen saturation, and urine output.[3]

Maternal vital signs typically do not change drastically until significant blood loss has occurred.[5]

Laboratory Evaluation

Laboratory evaluation should include (RCOG modified):

- FBC, coagulation, U&Es, LFTs
- Cross-match (4 units, FFP, PLT, cryoprecipitate)
- ECG, oximeter Foley catheter for urine volume
- Hemoglobin bedside testing
- Ionized calcium
- Potassium
- Transfusion targets
- Consider central and arterial lines.

In PPH, acute changes in hemoglobin or hematocrit will not accurately reflect blood loss.[5]

Accurate documentation is important for further clinical management, continuity of care and team work. In addition, inadequate documentation can contribute to the likelihood of there being medicolegal consequences.[5]

Transfuse Red Blood Cells, Platelets, Plasma

Recommendations are usually based upon expert opinion since there is no strong evidence from randomized trials, and these opinions are often extrapolated from data from studies in trauma patients. No consensus on the optimal ratio of blood product replacement; recommendations for RBC:FFP ratios vary widely (e.g. RBC:FFP: 1:1, 2:1, 3:2, 6:4).[3]

Women who received multiple transfusions after a vaginal delivery may receive (low-molecular-weight heparin (LMWH for prophylaxis against thrombotic events for 7–14 days postpartum.[3]

REFERENCES

1. Dahlke JD, Mendez-Figueroa H, Maggio L, et al. Prevention and management of postpartum hemorrhage: a comparison of 4 national guidelines. Am J Obstet Gynecol. 2015 Jul;213(1):76. e1-10.
2. French guidelines 2016.
3. Up To Date Oct 2017.
4. Maternal Health Division Ministry of Health and Family Welfare Government of India 2015.
5. ACOG GUIDE 2017.
6. RANZCOG Guide 2017.
7. WHO GUIDE 2012.
8. RCOG GUIDE 2016.
9. WOMAN Trial. Lancet. 2017.

Chapter 4

Massive Transfusion Protocol—What, How, and How Much?

Smita Mahapatra

BACKGROUND

Massive obstetric hemorrhage is a leading cause of maternal death and morbidity world-wise. In Asia and Africa, obstetric hemorrhage accounts for more than 30% of all maternal deaths in comparison to lower rates of maternal death in developed countries like 3.4% in United Kingdom and 11.4% in the United States. Transfusion therapy with red blood cells (RBC) and other blood products are the integral part in the management of major obstetrics hemorrhage.

WHAT?

Massive transfusion protocol (MTP) describes the process of management of blood transfusion requirements in major bleeding episodes, assisting the interactions of the treating clinicians and the blood bank, and ensuring judicious use of blood and blood components. MTP is the administration of 8–10 RBC units to an adult patient in less than 24 hours or as the acute administration of 4–5 RBC units in 1 hour. For patients identified as "low-risk" for transfusion, blood type testing for ABO system and Rhesus system only to be recommended. For patients deemed "moderate risk" for transfusion, testing for type and screen (T&S) is recommended. For patients considered to be "high-risk" for transfusion, a type and cross-match (T&C) to set-up RBC is recommended. MTP is required in massive hemorrhage in certain conditions like uterine atony, placenta accrete, placenta previa, placenta abruption, amniotic fluid embolism, and acute fatty liver.

METHODOLOGY

How?

Massive transfusion protocol should be immediately started in patients with active bleeding after 1–2 liters of blood loss aiming to reduce the maternal morbidity and mortality of the patient. The timing of initial transfusion of MTP ranges from 2–24 hours postdelivery. When a patient is at risk for uncontrolled bleeding, blood samples should be sent to the laboratory for disseminated intravascular coagulation (DIC) panel tests like prothrombin time (PT), partial thromboplastin time (PTT), fibrinogen, thrombin time, D-dimer, complete blood count (CBC), arterial blood gas (ABG), and to the blood bank for type and screen.

How Much?

Active MTP with initial MTP package comprises of the emergency release of 6 units of O-negative RBC, 4 units of plasma (AB plasma or thawed type of specific plasma), 1 apheresis platelet (PLT) unit. A patient in critical condition and with a limited supply of type-specific blood may require a change in the ABO or Rh types. A postmenopausal female patient may be switched from Rh-negative to Rh-positive blood. Additional MTP packages are provided as ordered by re-enactment of same scenario until the patient is stabilized and active bleeding is resolved. If international normalized ratio (INR) is more than 1.5 or PTT exceeds 60 seconds then 4 units of fresh frozen plasma (FFP) to be given. If PLT count is less than 50,000/cmm, 1 PLT should be transfused. The patient should be provided 10 packs of cryoprecipitate when the fibrinogen is less than 100 mg/dL to increase the fibrinogen. If the laboratory reports are not within normal limit or the active bleeding is ongoing the initial MTP pack to be repeated. Other hemostatic/blood replacement strategies like activated factor VII and antifibrinolytic agents can be considered. The role of recombinant activated factor VII (rFVIIa) to manage uncontrolled bleeding is unclear. However, it can be considered as a rescue therapy in patients with life-threatening bleeding that is unresponsive to standard hemostatic therapy. When rFVIIa is used, the recommended dose is 200 μg/kg initially followed by repeat dose of 100 μg/kg at 1 hour and 3 hours. Antifibrinolytic agents like tranexamic acid may be useful in bleeding complicated by fibrinolysis. Early administration of tranexamic acid in bleeding trauma patients has been shown to significantly reduce mortality. Besides, cell salvage can be extremely useful in unanticipated blood loss and in patients with rare blood groups. This strategy is generally reserved for massive blood loss in operation theaters as asepsis can be maintained easily. However, the relative contraindications such as a possibility of contamination with infected material and malignant cells should be considered. The MTP should be deactivated on the availability of normalize laboratory values and or with no evidence of ongoing bleeding. The physicians should consider the estimated blood loss (EBL) as part of the decision-making process for determining the total number of RBC units to be transfused from MTP. Transfusion of preordered cross-matched RBC can reduce the utilization of O-negative RBC inventory.

DISCUSSION

Massive transfusion protocols have a predefined ratio of RBCs, FFP/cryoprecipitate, and platelets units in each pack (e.g. 1:1:1 or 2:1:1 ratio) for transfusion. Once the patient is in the protocol, the blood bank ensures rapid and timely delivery of all blood components together to facilitate resuscitation. This reduces dependency on laboratory testing during the acute resuscitation phase and decreases the need for communication between the blood bank, laboratory, and physician.

There are certain limitations of MTP. First of all it is not standardized. The trigger for initiating the protocol as well as the optimum ratio of RBC:FFP: Platelets is controversial. Therefore practice varies from center to center. Secondly if MTP is triggered for a nonmassive blood loss situation, it may lead to wastage of blood products.

CONCLUSION

Massive transfusion protocol has been advocated as an essential tool for facilitating the early transfusion of sufficient volume and type of blood products for patients with massive obstetric hemorrhage. Management of massive loss requires a quick concerted team effort by many medical and paramedical members. Implementation of MTP has been shown to improve the timeliness of blood transfusion and to be cost effective (due to lower use of blood products). A hospital-based MTP specific to obstetric service can provide life-saving transfusion therapy for patients presenting with major obstetric hemorrhage.

Chapter 5

Nonpneumatic Antishock Garment

Gomathy Narayanan

INTRODUCTION

Nonpneumatic antishock garment (NASG) is used as a life-saving first aid device in uncontrollable postpartum hemorrhage (PPH). It controls bleeding, reverses shock, and stabilizes the patient's condition to enable safe transport to a center, which is equipped with comprehensive obstetric care facilities.

NONPNEUMATIC ANTISHOCK GARMENT (LIFE WRAP)

- It applies pressure on the legs and abdomen
- Blood returns to vital organs curbing internal bleed
- Stabilizes blood pressure (BP) until patient reaches appropriate hospital
- Easy to apply
- Application time takes less than 60 seconds in trained hands.

How does Nonpneumatic Antishock Garment Work?

- It is a first aid
- Controls bleeding through direct pressure
- Autotransfusion of blood in upward direction
- Ball in abdominal segment applies focused pressure to uterus
- Circumferential pressure on lower half of the body reduces the total vascular space
- Vital organs get increased blood supply and oxygenation
- Stabilization of patient during transport.

How does Nonpneumatic Antishock Garment Work?

The process of working of nonpneumatic antishock garment (NASG) is given Figure 5.1.

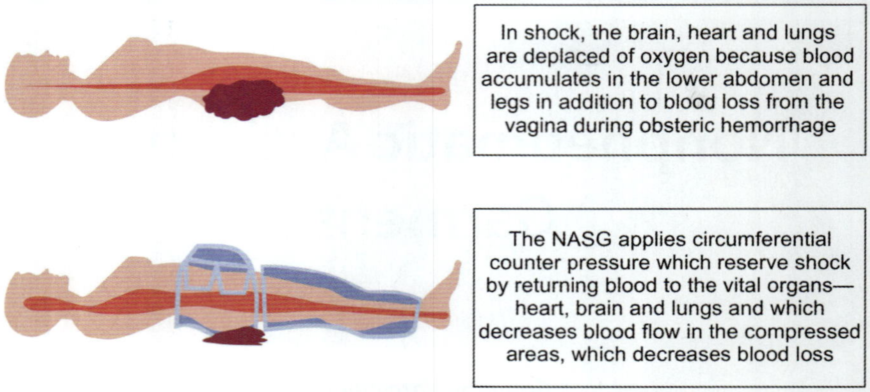

Fig. 5.1: Working of nonpneumatic antishock garment.

About Nonpneumatic Antishock Garment

- Nonpneumatic antishock garment is light weight (1500 g)
- Compression suit made of neoprene
- Six segments enclosing ankle, calves, thigh, pelvis, and abdomen
- Velcro fastenings to keep garment tight
- A small foam ball in the abdominal segment applies pressure on the uterus
- Markings on the sections show how to apply
- Correct tight application supplies 20–40 mm Hg of circumferential pressure to lower body effectively reversing hypovolemic shock
- Can be easily packed back into carry bag.

Applying Nonpneumatic Antishock Garment (Fig. 5.2)

Step 1

- Place NASG under the woman with the top at the level of lowest rib
- Close segment 1 tightly around ankle on both sides
- Snap it until you hear a sharp sound.

Step 2

- Close segment 2 around calf muscle
- Leave the knee joint free.

Step 3

- Apply segment 3 around the thighs.

Step 4

- Apply segment 4 all around the woman with the lower edge at the level of pubic bone.

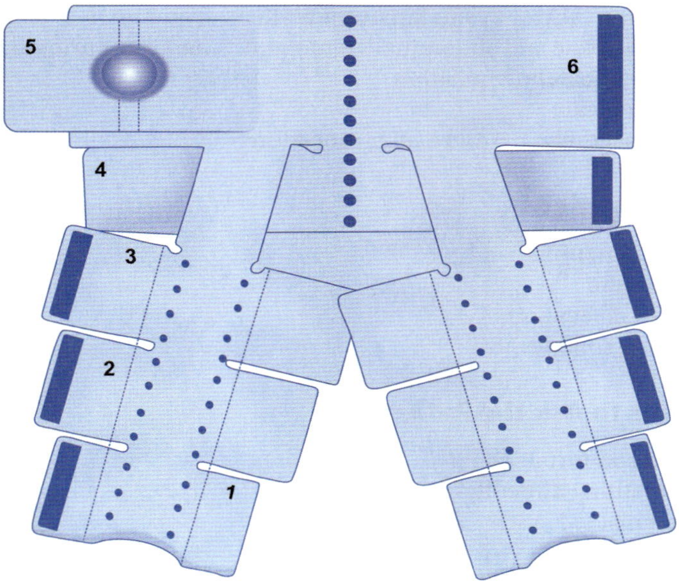

Fig. 5.2: Steps in nonpneumatic antishock garment (life wrap).

Step 5

- Place segment 5 with pressure ball directly over umbilicus
- Close the NSAG using segment 6
- Only one person should close segment 4 and 5
- Should not be too tight to restrict breathing.

Step 6

- Ensure patient is breathing normally after the application
- In case of uterine atony administer uterotonics and massage the uterus without removing the NASG
- Nonpneumatic antishock garment is flexible enough to allow the massaging.

Vaginal Procedures with Nonpneumatic Antishock Garment in situ

- Pelvic examination
- Lithotomy position
- Repair of episiotomy or perineal tear or vaginal laceration or cervical tear
- Manual removal of placenta (MRP)
- Bimanual compression
- Dilatation and curettage (D and C) or Dilatation and evacuation (D and E) or manual vacuum aspiration (MVA)

- Surgery with NASG in situ laparotomy (Keep segments 1, 2, and 3 in situ and open pelvic and abdominal segments 4, 5, and 6 just prior to incision)
- Steep Trendelenburg position
- Operate quickly
- Replace segment 4, 5 and 6 after procedure.

Special Situations

- Obese women
- Short stature
- Need for defecation
- Replacing soiled NASG.

Questions to Ask the Patient

- Are you comfortable?
- Any breathing difficulty?
- Is it hot inside NASG?
- Do you feel itch?

When to Remove Nonpneumatic Antishock Garment?

- Patient must be stable for 2 hours
- Bleeding less than 50 mL/hour
- Pulse less than 100 beats per minute (BPM)
- Systolic BP 90–100 mm Hg
- Hemoglobin (Hb) more than 7G%
- Patient conscious and aware.

How to Remove Nonpneumatic Antishock Garment?

- Remove segment 1 and wait for 15 minutes
- Check pulse and BP
- *If pulse rate increases more than 20 BPM or BP falls by 20 mm Hg*: Reapply segment 1
- If vitals stable remove segment 2
- Follow same principles till removal of segment 6.

Do not remove NASG before all vital signs are restored Early removal of NASG can be dangerous or even fatal.

Caution

- If BP falls by 20 mm Hg or pulse increases by 20 BPM after removal of any segment, rapidly replace all segments
- Consider need for crystalloids or Blood
- If recurrent bleeding, determine source and arrest.

Storing Nonpneumatic Antishock Garment

- Clean NASG with running water and disinfectant and dry
- Keep folded NASG in a clear plastic bag
- Store NASG in a place where it is visible and accessible
- Always store at the same place
- Ensure everyone knows place of storage
- Storage place should be displayed prominently
- The referral center must send a replacement NASG after receiving the patient
- Relative contraindications
- Cardiac failure
- Preexisting mitral stenosis or pulmonary edema
- Advanced pregnancy with live fetus (APH)
- Abdominal evisceration
- Open pelvic fracture.

Principles to be Observed

- One person alone can apply NASG
- Two persons needed when patient is unconscious
- Urine output should be measured
- Ensure airway protection and prevent aspiration
- Ensure one on one nursing care.

Advantages of Nonpneumatic Antishock Garment

- About 50–78% reduction in blood loss
- About 50–55% reduction in maternal mortality and related morbidity
- World Health Organization (WHO) includes NASG in recommendations
- Cost effective
- Reusable.

The experts,[1,2] who pioneered the device is of the opinion that it can reduce death at child birth by over 50%. According to Professor Miller, it is a very potent first aid device which could have a huge impact on reducing the maternal morbidity and mortality. (Fig.5.3)

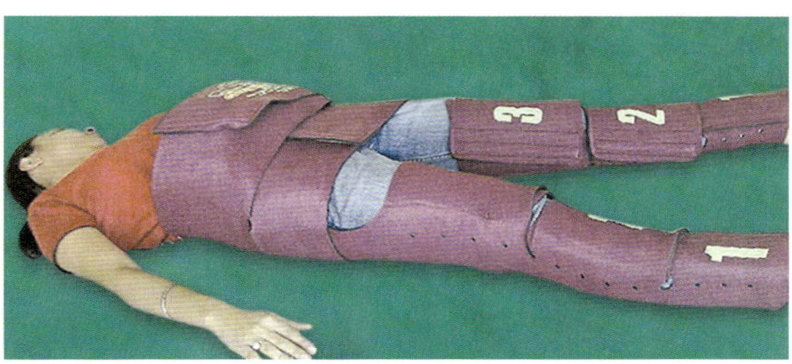

Fig. 5.3: Impact on reducing the maternal morbidity and mortality.

WHO recommends NASG in low resource settings especially, because it is cost-effective and reusable. It has been used successfully in over 6,000 women in 6 countries. In UK and USA, it is being used in remote rural areas and in Jehovah's Witness women who decline blood transfusion. In African countries such as Zambia and Zimbabwe, it is being used in urban centers as well. The Tamil Nadu Government has made NASG available in all health centers and also in ambulances.

The method of application of NASG, cleaning, storing, and its use in special situations are demonstrated in the YouTube video titled, "Saving mothers' lives and NASG training video" (www.youtube.com/watch?v=tSGC7VHoN_E)

REFERENCES

1. Morris J, Meyer C, Fathalla MF, et al. Treating Uterine Atony with the NASG in Egypt. African Journal of Midwifery and Women's Health. 2011;5(1):37-42.
2. Ojengbede O, Galadanci H, Morhason-Bello IO, et al. The Non-pneumatic Anti-Shock Garment for Postpartum Haemorrhage in Nigeria. African Journal of Midwifery and Women's Health. 2011;5(3):135-9.

Chapter 6

Uterine Tamponade: The Newer Methods, Controversies and Consensus

H Samartha Ram

INTRODUCTION

As per the World Health Organization (WHO) estimate, 287,000 maternal deaths occurred globally in the year 2010. Low resource countries like India (19%) and Nigeria (14%) accounted for one-third (96,000) of global burden. In India, postpartum hemorrhage (PPH) was the leading cause, and in majority of women, atonic PPH was the cause. Even though some risk factors like obstructed prolonged labor, accidental hemorrhage, and big babies are known to cause atonic PPH, it is not very clear why some women develop atonic PPH and why some women do not. For the same reason, this problem cannot be predictable. The only management strategy even today is "watchful expectancy" and to act immediately when the problem arises. Simpler techniques like uterine massage, uterotonic drugs, and uterine packing and balloon tamponade can be practiced in low-resource settings. Techniques like B-Lynch suturing, stepwise devascularization, internal iliac ligation and uterine artery embolization are available only at higher medical centers. These higher techniques are not within the reach of every parturient woman when simpler techniques fail. In low-resource settings, unpredictable sudden massive bleeding makes it difficult to organize competent manpower, compatible blood and transport to higher medical center. Many times, mothers die on roads while being transported to higher medical centers due to hypovolemic shock. In some women, the speed with which the hemorrhage kills the mother is so rapid that the usually quoted first 1 hour or 2 hours as "golden hours" is missing. Sometimes women succumb to death just within 1–1.5 hours after the onset of bleeding. The rapidity with which some women slip into coagulation failure and multiorgan dysfunction syndrome from hemorrhagic shock is alarming. Because of these complex reasons, the maternal mortality is not coming down in low-resource settings. There is much need for a simpler and sure technique which can stop bleeding, or at least stop bleeding temporarily to buy some time to tide over the crisis.

CONCEPT

Creating negative pressure inside the uterine cavity results in shrinking of uterus which can assist the natural physiological process of contraction and retraction to stop atonic PPH.

METHODS

Sixteen singleton pregnant women who had normal vaginal deliveries and 4 women who underwent cesarean sections, and who developed atonic PPH, and who did not respond for routine methods were included in this study. All the women received 10 units of oxytocin intramuscular (IM) at the appearance of anterior shoulder, 5 units of intravenous oxytocin after the delivery of placenta, and then the uterine massage. Injection carboprost 125 µg IM was also given when the bleeding did not stop.

DESCRIPTION OF UTERINE VACUUM RETRACTION SYSTEM

It consists of:

- *Uterine retraction cannulas:* Five different sizes (25 cm-L×2.4 cm-D, 25 cm-L×2.0 cm-D, 25 cm-L×1.4 cm-D, 14 cm-L×2.0 cm-D, and 14 cm-L×1.4 cm-D) are made to match different cervical dilatations and for different applications (Fig. 6.1). There is uterine angle, and there are perforations on fundal and cervical portions. Perforations on fundal portion are large and longitudinal, and on cervical portion, they are round and small (Fig. 6.1).
- Thick walled, not easily collapsible flexible plastic suction tube.
- High vacuum suction machine, or vacuum suction pump which can produce a negative pressure up to 650 mm Hg. within 1 minute.

In Case of Vaginal Delivery

Two sizes are made for this purpose. Bigger size (2.4 cm-D) is designed for massive atonic PPH (Fig. 6.1A). Smaller size (2.0 cm-D) is designed for prophylactic application in high-risk women for atonic PPH (Fig. 6.1B). Usually, the smaller size is used first. If bleeding is massive, and if the cannula is not retaining inside the uterus, then we should go for the bigger size.

When bleeding did not stop by routine medical measures, under 30 mg pentazocine, and 0.6 mg of atropine intravenous analgesia (needs no sedation if cooperative), women should be kept in lithotomy position, and the bladder catheterized. Under good source of light, with wide blade vaginal speculum application, the genital tract should be explored to exclude traumatic PPH and to confirm uterine atony. Blood clots should be removed from uterine cavity by bimanual compression. The anterior lip of cervix should be grasped with sponge holding forceps. The nipple of the cannula should be firmly fitted to

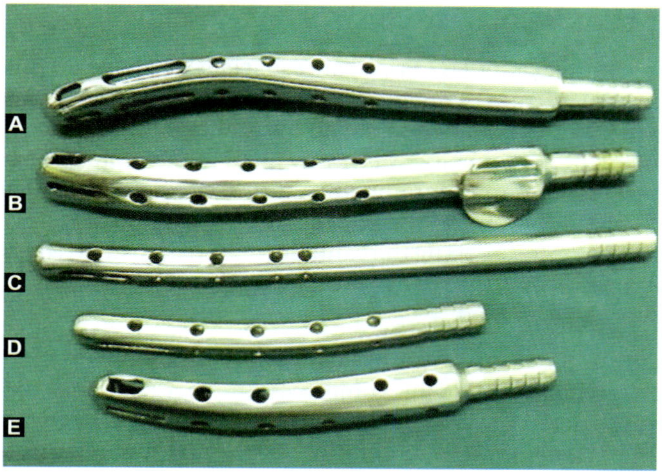

Figs. 6.1A to E: Different sizes of cannulas to match different cervical dilatations, and for different applications. A, B and C are vaginal cannulas. 'A' is meant for massive atonic postpartum hemorrhage, 'B' for prophylactic application, and 'C' for bleeding after medical termination of pregnancy. 'D' and 'E' are designed for use during cesarean section.

one end of suction tube and the other end is connected to suction machine. Uterine end of the cannula should be inserted into the uterine cavity up to the level of fundus. Sponge holder and speculum should be removed. The left palm supporting the fundus per abdomen, right fingers grasping the outer end of the cannula, cannula should be pushed gently up to the fundus. Keeping the cannula in this position (to prevent slipping out), suction machine should be put on and a negative pressure of 650 mm Hg should be applied for 10 minutes. Then the suction machine should be put off. This makes the cannula get fixed in this position due to sucking of soft cervical tissues into the perforations on cervical portion of the cannula. After first application of negative pressure, negative pressure should be applied for 10 minutes at every hour for 3 hours, or whenever the bleeding recurs.

Twenty units of oxytocin drip in 5% dextrose, 40–60 drops/min was run throughout the procedure. The cannula was kept in position as long as the obstetrician feels the threat of recurrence of bleeding, even up to 24 hours.

Cannula removal: After the procedure, if we try to pull out the cannula, it will not come out easily. The temporary adhesions developed due to sucking of soft cervical tissues into perforations of the cervical portion of the cannula should be released by gentle finger manipulation. After this, the cannula will come out easily. We should not try to remove the cannula immediately after application of negative pressure. Cannula should be removed at least 30–60 minutes after last application of negative pressure. If roughly pulled, the cervix may get injured and may start bleeding.

In Case of Cesarean Section

Two sizes of shorter cannulas (14 cm) are especially designed for this purpose. Big size cannula (20 mm diameter) is meant for dilated cervix, and the small size cannula (1.4 cm diameter) is meant for undilated cervix (Figs. 6.1D and E). One end of the suction tube was firmly fitted to the nipple of the cannula. The other end was inserted through the uterine wound and brought outside the vagina. The outer end of the suction tube should be connected to the suction machine. After keeping the cannula in proper position (tip at the level of fundus), and keeping the cut edges of the uterine wound together, negative pressure should be applied.

Prophylactic application of cannula during vaginal delivery: Prophylactic application is recommended for women who are at risk for developing atonic PPH, like obstructed prolonged labor, accidental hemorrhage, pregnancy-induced hypertension, anemia complicating pregnancy, and multifetal pregnancy. For this purpose, a especially designed cannula with wings (B) is advised. Wings are meant for supporting the tight packing of the episiotomy wound with surgical pad to minimize blood loss.

Before the delivery of the baby itself, the vacuum suction cannula system should be organized and kept ready (connecting the nipple of the cannula to suction tube, and connecting the suction tube to the suction machine) (Fig. 6.2). After the delivery of the baby, a wide blade vaginal speculum should be applied, and 4–5 cm of anterior lip of cervix should be grasped with sponge holding forceps. After the delivery of placenta, mild traction should be applied on cervix by gently pulling the sponge holder, and then the uterine end of the cannula should be inserted into the uterine cavity up to the level of fundus. Left palm supporting the fundus per abdomen feels the position of cannula.

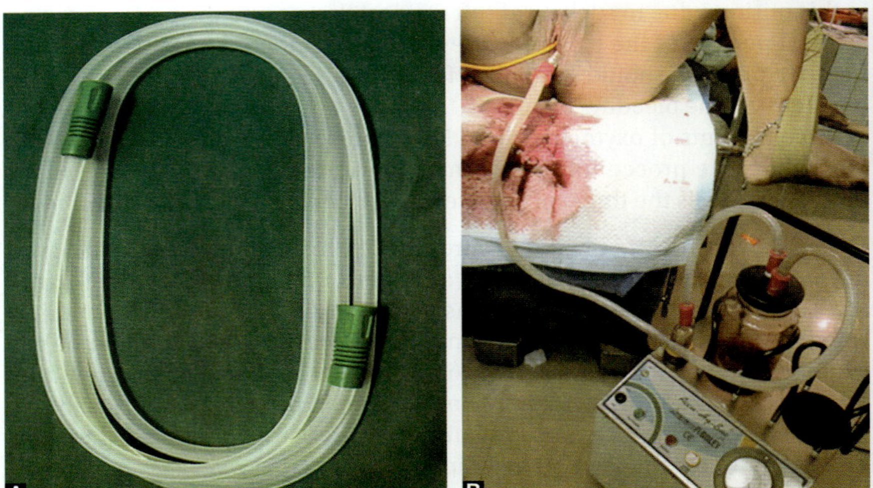

Figs. 6.2A and B: (A) Thick walled (not easily collapsible) flexible plastic suction tube; (B) Vacuum suction cannula in position connected to suction machine.

This helps to avoids perforation. The cannula should be held in this position, and a negative pressure of 650 mm Hg should be applied by putting on the suction machine. This helps to fix the cannula in this position and also stops bleeding.

DIFFERENT SIZES OF CANNULAS

Negative pressure should be applied for 20 minutes and then suction machine is put off. Machine can be put on whenever there is recurrence of bleeding. If there is difficulty in inserting one size of the cannula, downsizing can be done. Uterotonic drugs may also be given depending on the need.

MECHANISM—HOW IT ACTS

When negative pressure is applied, the soft cervical tissues around the cervical portion of the cannula get sucked into the perforations resulting in closed uterine cavity. Further application of suction results in firm contraction and retraction of uterus on the surface of the cannula. This assists the natural physiological process of contraction and retraction to stop atonic bleeding (Fig. 6.3).

RESULTS OF OUR STUDY

Complete cessation of bleeding which was associated with contraction and firm retraction of uterus was observed in all women within 4 minutes after initiation of procedure. None of the women had recurrence of bleeding after 3 hours after initiation of procedure. All the women were clinically stable during the procedure. The amount of blood collected in suction bottle ranged from

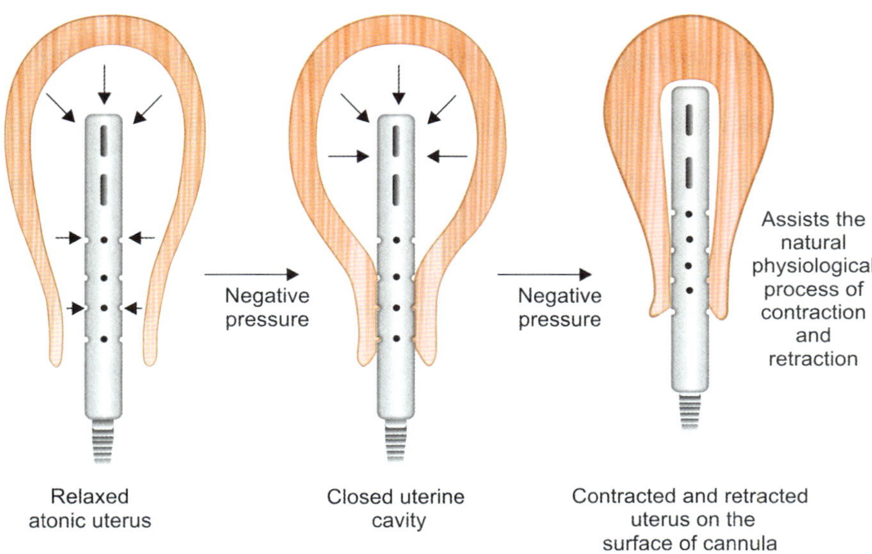

Fig. 6.3: Mechanisms how negative pressure inside the uterine cavity stops atonic bleeding.

150 mL to 250 mL. At cesarean section, we could observe contraction and firm retraction of uterus with the formation of rugosities on the surface of uterus.

DISCUSSION

In our present study, vacuum retraction could stop bleeding in all women within 4 minutes after the initiation of negative pressure. Few cases were reported (verbal communication) that the PPH cannula system could stop bleeding even in women with disseminated intravascular coagulation (DIC). Currently, the balloon tamponade is being widely advocated as an affordable alternative to blood loss management in severe atonic PPH refractory to uterotonic therapy. In this technique, the water-filled balloon expands the uterine cavity and applies constant pressure (more than the systolic blood pressure) on sinusoids to stop bleeding. The mechanism of action in this technique is against the natural physiological mechanism of contraction and retraction. It requires sometimes to organize this balloon tamponade system. This technique cannot be used when tamponade test is negative. When the woman is bleeding profusely, even this few minutes time is very precious and critical.

In contrast, the mechanism involved with vacuum constriction and retraction assists the natural physiological process of contraction and retraction (Fig. 6.3). As the blood circulation to uterus is not interfered, the uterotonic drugs continue to act and maintain the process of contraction and retraction. Blood collected in the uterine cavity get sucked and collected into the suction bottle and helps to measure the blood loss correctly. As this procedure needs little time and minimal skills, even maternity nurses can be trained and the bleeding can be stopped without any delay.

Mechanism--how it Works?

The mechanism of negative pressure inside the uterine cavity is given in Figure 6.3.

CONCLUSION

Vacuum retraction of uterus with SR cannula is a simple, cost effective, can stop bleeding within 4 minutes, avoids laparotomy, preserves fertility function, and prevents maternal death in low-resource settings. Prophylactic application of cannula in high-risk pregnancies further helps to reduce the incidence of atonic PPH. Its utilization in cases of inherited coagulopathies of pregnancy and DIC has to be further explored with a larger sample size.

This paper got prestigious Senior category **'FOGSI CORION AWARD'** for the year 2017 to be presented at AICOG Bhubaneswar.

This paper was awarded FOGSI Dr CS Dawn prize at AICOG-2015, Chennai.

This paper was awarded KFOG President Gold medal for the year 2015.

This article was published in IOSR Journal of Dental and Medical Sciences (IOSR-JDMS) in November 2014.

This cannula got patent registered in September 2015.

Chapter 7

Management of Postpartum Hemorrhage: Where Do We Go Wrong?

Sabaratnam Arulkumaran

"*Too little, too late*" has been highlighted in successive confidential inquiries into maternal deaths in the United Kingdom. Key elements where we go wrong are not considering the woman may be anemic at the onset, that her blood volume is related to her body weight, poor assessment of blood loss and not following a stepwise progression of management to stem the hemorrhage and manage the woman's blood loss appropriately. The stepwise rapid succession of medical followed by surgical interventions can stop or minimize the bleeding and correct the blood loss and prevent the cascade of events that lead to massive blood loss, hysterectomy, admission to intensive care unit (ICU) and deaths and is tackled by the use of the mnemonic "HEMOSTASIS". Give oxygen, adequate fluids, blood and blood products. No response to oxytocin or, ergometrine warrants infusion of oxytocin to keep the uterus contracted to allow clotting of uterine vessels. Next step is bimanual uterine massage and prostaglandins (parenteral PGF or misoprostol PGE1 orally or sublingually). Blood loss could be about 70 mL/minute when the uterus relaxes and hence a 14-gauge needle to give fluids rapidly should be used X 2 lines. Tranexamic acid, an antithrombolytic prevents the clot from lysing. An antishock garment, which squeezes the blood into the circulation and also has a compressive effect on the uterus, could be tried. Consumptive coagulopathy, lack of clotting factors, activation of fibrinolysis, large volumes of fluids, metabolic acidosis and hypothermia aggravate the situation and are controlled by fibrinogen and clotting factors. Shock is proportionate to blood loss—mild 15%, moderate 30%, and severe 45%. Transfusion of one unit packed red blood cells to unit plasma as opposed to four packed cells to one unit plasma results in a 60–70% reduction in mortality in war injury victims—same principle after blood loss of more than 2 L of blood loss is useful. Freeze dried fibrinogen concentrate that can be reconstituted may be an alternative. Platelet transfusion may be needed but this is rare. Failure to arrest hemorrhage by medical therapy should be followed by a "Tamponade test". It will only work when there is no coagulopathy. Sengstaken, Rusch, or

Cooke's catheter can be inserted into the uterus and filled with warm saline/water bleeding completely stops. If bleeding stops the balloon can be taken out in 6 hours. Patient should have broad-spectrum antibiotics and an oxytocin infusion. Vital parameters, fundal height and bleeding per vagina should be monitored. If the test is going to be effective it will be known within 5 minutes. If the tamponade fails to stop the bleeding, a laparotomy should be performed and compression sutures (B-Lynch or 2–5 vertical) should be employed. Failure of compression sutures should lead to systematic devascularization by tying the infundibulopelvic and uterine vessels and/or anterior branch of the internal iliacs. Arterial embolization using radiological guidance can be tried where facilities exist. Failure to arrest hemorrhage or deterioration of general condition of the patient should prompt subtotal or total hysterectomy. The recent research—WOMAN trial consisting of 20,000 women has informed us that the use of a clot stabilizer tranexamic acid would reduce the maternal deaths by 30% if administered within 3 hours of the postpartum hemorrhage (PPH). The long-acting heat stable Duratocin (half-life approximately 80 minutes) may be better than Syntocinon which has a half-life of 4 minutes. The CHAMPION trial that would recruit 30,000 women may revolutionize the medications we may give. If blood transfusion is needed, one packed cells to one plasma compared with four red cells to plasma may help to save many lives and reduce morbidity. The management of placenta accreta may be best with a "Triple P procedure" pioneered at St George's Hospital may find more acceptance as it excises the placenta with part of myometrium and allows reconstruction and retention of the uterus. If hysterectomy is contemplated delivery of baby should be from above the placental site, no oxytocin, nonremoval of placenta and ligation of new vessels from bladder base before starting hysterectomy. New regimen of drugs and simple technology may help many women to survive and retain their uterus and reduce overall morbidity. We go wrong if we do not follow the simple principles.

Chapter 8

Heart Disease in Pregnancy: A Cardiologist Message to Obstetricians

SN Routray

ABSTRACT

Cardiovascular diseases are being increasingly encountered in clinical practice by medical practitioners. A thorough understanding of the normal physiology of pregnancy and of the various cardiovascular diseases in pregnancy is imperative to the successful management of such patients
Keywords: Pregnancy, hemodynamics, cardiovascular disorders

INTRODUCTION

Cardiovascular disease (CVD) affects 0.2–4% of pregnant women but account for one-third of all pregnancy-related deaths.[1] The maternal mortality in CVD patients is about 1% which is 100 times more than the normal pregnant population. Congenital heart disease (CHD) comprises the largest category of CVD in the West while rheumatic heart disease (RHD) constitutes 30% of CVD in pregnancy in developing countries.[2] While modern medicine enables an increasing number of CHD patients to attain childbearing age, ischemic heart disease incidence is also rising due to advancing maternal age and risk factors (smoking, obesity, diabetes and hypertension). The inextricable consequences of the illness on the fetus further compound the magnitude of the problem demanding the attention of all health care personnel involved in maternal and child care.

The hemodynamic changes occurring in pregnancy impose a significant load on the diseased heart. Blood volume rises by about 50% disproportionate to rise in RBC mass leading to anemia of pregnancy. Cardiac output (CO) rises mostly on account of rise in stroke volume and reaches a peak at the end of second trimester making it the most susceptible time for cardiac decompensation. Reduction of systemic vascular resistance causes blood pressure (BP) to fall until the same stage and return to prepregnancy levels by term. An increase in the level of clotting factors coupled with stasis due to compression of inferior vena cava (IVC) by the gravid uterus makes pregnancy a hypercoagulable state. During labor, pain, anxiety and uterine contractions result in an increased BP and increase in cardiac output up to 75%. An average of 300–500 mL of blood loss occurs during delivery. In the postpartum period, decompression of IVC and autotransfusion results in a sudden surge of venous return resulting in a 60–80% rise in CO which may precipitate pulmonary edema. The hemodynamic changes return to baseline by 2–4 weeks following delivery. Such drastic hemodynamic alterations may result in signs and symptoms similar to heart disease even in healthy patients. Dyspnea and fatigue are common symptoms. Raised jugular venous pressure (JVP), mild peripheral edema, S3 and systolic flow murmurs are physiological findings. Exertional chest pain, orthopnea, paroxysmal nocturnal dyspnea, loud systolic murmurs and diastolic murmurs are red flag signs indicative of cardiac pathology.

Individual cardiac lesions impact pregnancy differently with mortality varying from less than 1% in New York Heart Association class I–II patients to 6.8% in class III–IV. Conditions considered contraindications to pregnancy include severe pulmonary hypertension of any etiology, severe fixed obstructive cardiac lesions, NYHA class III–IV heart failure, left ventricular ejection fraction (LVEF) less than 40%, prior peripartum cardiomyopathy (PPCM), dilated unstable aorta of 40–45 mm or above, or severe cyanosis. The cardiac disease in pregnancy (CARPREG) score system is comprised of four clinical features—prior cardiac event, NYHA class III/IV or cyanosis, valvular or outflow tract obstruction and LV dysfunction with 1 point for each .The maternal event rate for a cumulative score of 0,1 and less than 1 is 5%, 27% and 75%, respectively.[3]

LOW-RISK LESIONS

Left to right shunts including atrial septal defect (ASD), ventricular septal defect (VSD), or a patent ductus artery (PDA) generally reduce in severity during pregnancy due to fall in peripheral vascular resistance. In the absence of pulmonary hypertension (PH), these lesions are well tolerated. Paradoxical embolism is a concern in ASD and aspirin use should be considered for prevention. Isolated pulmonary stenosis (PS) is well tolerated. If severe PS leads to right heart failure, balloon valvuloplasty should be considered, preferably in second trimester. Chronic regurgitant lesions are well tolerated due to fall in systemic vascular resistance and shortening of diastole [for aortic regurgitation (AR)]. Rheumatic and myxomatous valve degeneration are the principal etiologies of severe mitral regurgitation (MR). Symptomatic heart failure should be managed with afterload reducing agents like dihydropyridine calcium channel blockers (CCBs) and diuretics. Angiotensin-converting enzyme (ACE) inhibitors and angiotensin II receptor blockers (ARBs) are strictly contraindicated in pregnancy.

MODERATE RISK LESIONS

Rheumatic mitral stenosis is the most common valve lesion in women of childbearing age. Exertional breathlessness, pulmonary edema or atrial fibrillation may lead to de novo detection of MS in pregnancy. Fetal outcome is also adversely affected with marked increased incidence of preterm delivery, intrauterine growth restriction (IUGR), low-birth weight babies and fetal death. Mild MS remains mostly asymptomatic. Moderate to severe MS is managed with diuretics, beta blockers and anticoagulation (for atrial fibrillation). Refractory cases are treated with balloon mitral valvuloplasty preferably in second trimester to avoid teratogenic effects of radiation. Cardiopulmonary bypass is associated with fetal mortality of 20–30% and hence, mitral valve replacement is rarely performed in pregnancy.[4]

Aortic stenosis is due to a congenital bicuspid valve or rheumatic. Severe AS presents with dyspnea, angina or syncope. The medical therapy is limited and includes bed rest and cautious diuresis. For persistent symptoms, percutaneous balloon valvuloplasty should be considered in suitable valves and valve replacement only in refractory cases as a last resort. Coarctation of aorta (repaired and unrepaired) may be complicated with hypertension, heart failure, angina and aortic dissection. Poorly controlled hypertension may lead to rupture of intracranial aneurysms and must be controlled with β-blockers as the drug of choice. Marfan's syndrome is associated with an increased risk of aortic rupture or dissection especially in the postpartum period. Use of β blockers, serial echocardiography to monitor aortic root size and termination of pregnancy or aortic root replacement for progressive root dilation are recommended.

HIGH-RISK LESIONS

Pregnancy is not advised in these cases and if it occurs, termination of pregnancy should be strongly considered. Eisenmenger's syndrome is associated with a maternal mortality of 30–50% and fetal mortality of 50% in surviving mothers. Most of the complications occur in early postpartum period with thromboembolic disease being a prime contributor. Treatment includes anticoagulation, oxygen and pulmonary vasodilators. In uncorrected congenital cyanotic heart disease such as tetralogy of Fallot (TOF), right to left shunt increases leading to deepening of cyanosis. Maternal oxygen saturation less than 85% translates to less than 12% rate of live births. Pregnancy in repaired TOF is well tolerated although severe pulmonary regurgitation (PR) is a bad prognostic factor. Heart failure of any etiology with EF less than 40% or class III–IV symptoms is associated with extremely poor maternal and fetal outcomes.

ACQUIRED CARDIOVASCULAR DISORDERS IN PREGNANCY

Hypertension in pregnancy is defined as a BP less than 140/90 mm Hg and is classified as gestational, chronic and preeclampsia with/without preexisting hypertension. Chronic hypertension is associated with 50% excess risk of small for gestational age neonate. Maternal and fetal mortality associated with preeclampsia and eclampsia is significant with evidence of substandard care in 64% of deaths.[5] The evidence regarding hypertension treatment is tenuous. BP above 150–160/100–110 mm Hg should be treated to prevent maternal end-organ damage. Oral methyldopa, labetalol, hydralazine and nifedipine are recommended while ACEI and ARBs are contraindicated. Intravenous labetalol, hydralazine or sodium nitroprusside may be used in hypertensive emergencies.

Peripartum cardiomyopathy (PPCM) is defined as new-onset idiopathic LV systolic dysfunction in the interval between the last month of pregnancy and the first 5 months postpartum. Although the etiology is unknown, older maternal age, multiparity, multifetal gestations, hypertensive disorders during pregnancy and low socioeconomic status are considered risk factors. 2 year mortality is about 9–15%. About 50% of women recover LV function usually within 6 months of delivery.[6] Treatment includes standard drugs for heart failure except ACEI and ARB during pregnancy. Bromocriptine and IV immunoglobulin have shown promising results in small studies. The risk of recurrence is 30–50% and residual LV dysfunction is a contraindication for future pregnancy.

Acute myocardial infarction in pregnancy is rare and more often due to spontaneous coronary artery dissection, in situ thrombosis or coronary spasm than obstructive coronary artery disease. Majority of patients are more than 30 years of age with a high incidence of conventional risk factors and the predominant presentation is STEMI.[7] Treatment is the same as nonpregnant women including use of percutaneous coronary intervention. Thrombolytic therapy is relatively contraindicated.

PROSTHETIC HEART VALVES

Women with well-functioning bioprosthetic valves and normal hemodynamics may safely undertake a pregnancy perhaps at the cost of accelerated structural deterioration of the valve.[8] Mechanical valves are associated with an increased incidence of thromboembolic events during pregnancy and hence, effective anticoagulation is critical. Warfarin is associated with embryopathy and miscarriage during 6–12 weeks of pregnancy. The current ACC/AHA guidelines recommend continuation of warfarin during the first trimester if required dose is less than 5 mg/day and replacement with dose adjusted continuous IV UFH or subcutaneous LMWH if required dose is higher. Warfarin is also to be replaced with UFH before a planned vaginal delivery. In both bioprosthetic and mechanical valves, aspirin (75–100 mg) is recommended in second and third trimesters.[9]

CONCLUSION

Heart disease in pregnancy encompasses a myriad of disorders with varying outcomes ranging from uneventful to lethal. The double jeopardy to maternal and child health necessitates meticulous care throughout pregnancy and beyond by a team including obstetricians, physicians and cardiologists to optimize outcomes and improve the quality of life of the female cardiac patients.

KEY POINTS

- Pregnancy may not be advisable for women with certain high-risk heart disorders (e.g. pulmonary hypertension, coarctation of the aorta if uncorrected or accompanied by an aneurysm, Marfan syndrome with aortic root diameter of more than 4.5 cm, severe symptomatic aortic stenosis, severe mitral stenosis, bicuspid aortic valve with ascending aorta more than 50 mm, a single ventricle with impaired systolic function, cardiomyopathy, NYHA class III or IV heart failure).
- Treat heart failure and arrhythmias during pregnancy as for nonpregnant patients, except avoid certain drugs (e.g. warfarin, ACE inhibitors, ARBs, aldosterone antagonists, thiazide diuretics, certain antiarrhythmics such as amiodarone).
- Treat most pregnant patients who have atrial fibrillation with standard or low molecular weight heparin.
- Indications for endocarditis prophylaxis for pregnant patients with a structural heart disorder are the same as those for other patients.

REFERENCES

1. Regitz ZV, Blomstrom LC, Borghi C, et al. ESC Guidelines on the management of cardiovascular diseases during pregnancy: The Task Force on the Management of Cardiovascular Diseases during Pregnancy of the European Society of Cardiology (ESC). Eur Heart J. 2011;32(24):3147-97.
2. Sliwa K, Libhaber E, Elliot C, et al. Spectrum of cardiac disease in a low resource cohort in South Africa. Heart. 2014;100(24):1967-74.
3. Siu SC, Sermer M, Colman JM, et al. Prospective multicenter study of pregnancy outcomes in women with heart disease. Circulation. 2001;104:515-21.
4. Silversides CK, Colman JM, Sermer M, et al. Cardiac risk in pregnant women with rheumatic mitral stenosis. Am J Cardiol. 2003;91:1382-5.
5. Cantwell R, Clutton-Brock T, Cooper G, et al. Centre for Maternal and Child Enquiries (CMACE): Saving mothers' lives: reviewing maternal deaths to make motherhood safer: 2006-08. The Eighth Report on Confidential Enquiries into Maternal Deaths in the United Kingdom. BJOG. 2011;118 Suppl 1:1-203.
6. McNamara DM, Elkayam U, Alharethi R, et al. for the IPAC Investigators. Clinical outcomes for peripartum cardiomyopathy in North America: results of the IPAC Study (Investigations of Pregnancy-associated Cardiomyopathy). J Am Coll Cardiol. 2015;66:905-14.
7. Roth A, Elkayam U. Acute myocardial infarction associated with pregnancy. J Am Coll Cardiol. 2008;52:171-80.
8. Elkayam, Bitar F. Valvular heart disease and pregnancy: part II: prosthetic valves. J Am Coll Cardiol. 2005;46:403-8.
9. Nishimura RA, Otto CM, Bonow RO, et al. 2014 AHA/ACC guideline for the management of patients with valvular heart disease: executive summary: a report of the American College of Cardiology/American Heart Association Task Force on Practice Guidelines. J Am Coll Cardiol. 2014;63:2438-88.

Chapter 9

Jaundice in Pregnancy—Maternal and Fetal Outcome

Mamta Rath Datta

INTRODUCTION

Abnormal liver tests occur in 3–5% of pregnancies, with many potential causes that may either be peculiar to pregnancy or may be coincidental to pregnancy. Management of a pregnant woman with jaundice poses a clinical challenge considering the need to optimize both the maternal and fetal outcome (Flowchart 8.1).

CAUSES OF JAUNDICE IN PREGNANCY (TABLE 8.1)

- Causes unique to pregnancy
  - Intrahepatic cholestasis of pregnancy (ICP)
  - Acute fatty liver of pregnancy (AFLP)
  - Preeclampsia—eclampsia and hemolysis, elevated liver enzymes and low platelets (HELLP) syndrome
  - Severe hyperemesis gravidarum (HG)
- Causes coincidental to pregnancy
  - Hepatic causes
    - Acute viral hepatitis
    - Drug induced
    - Chronic hepatitis
      - Viral
      - Autoimmune
    - Wilson's disease
    - Cirrhosis of liver
  - Prehepatic causes
- Hemolytic jaundice—hemolytic anemia, mismatched blood transfusion, malaria, and *Clostridium welchii* infection
  - Posthepatic causes
    - Common bile duct stone/strictures

Flowchart 8.1: Approach to a pregnant lady with jaundice

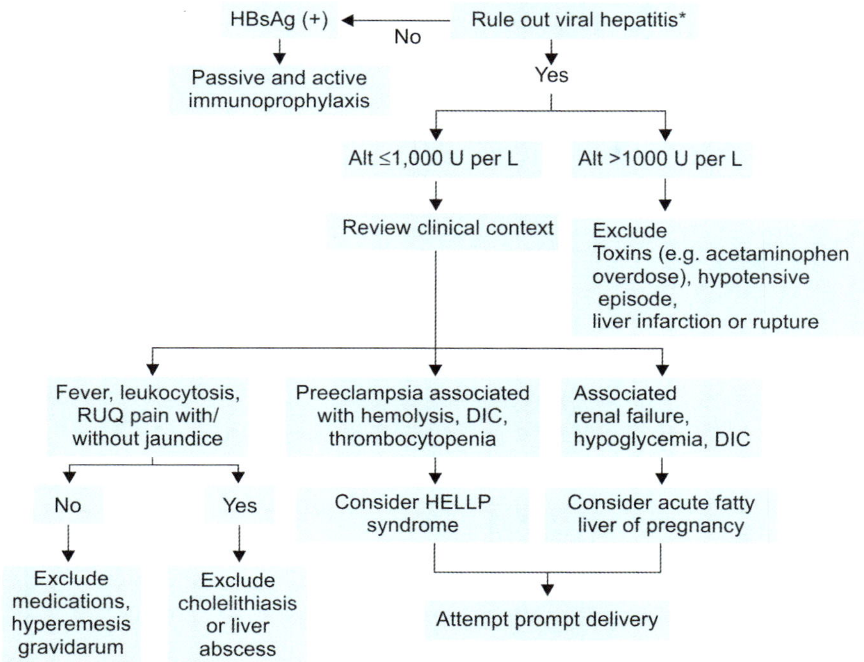

*Recommended serologic tests: Hepatitis A IgM, hepatitis B surgace antigen and hepatitis B core antibody, hepatitis C antibodies, Cytomegalovirus Igm, herpes simplex virus Igm, and Epstein-Barr virus Igm.

(HBsAg: hepatitis B virus surface antigen; ALT; alanine transaminase; RUQ: right upper quadrant; DIC: disseminated intravascular coagulation; HELLP: hemolysis, elevated liver enzymes and low platelets; IgM: immunoglobulin M)

(*Source:* Hunt CM, Sharara AI. Liver Disease in Pregnancy. Am Fam Physician. 1999;59(4):829-36).

INTRAHEPATIC CHOLESTASIS OF PREGNANCY

Intrahepatic cholestasis of pregnancy occurs in the late second or third trimester and has a prevalence of about 1/1,000–1/10,000. ICP is also more common in women of advanced maternal age, multiparous women and in women with a personal history of cholestasis with oral contraceptive use.[1] The prognosis is usually good, but it is associated with increased fetal morbidity and mortality, particularly from chronic placental insufficiency, preterm labor, fetal distress, and intrauterine death.[2]

The etiology is multifactorial. Mutations in the phospholipid translocator known as the ATP cassette transporter B4 (ABCB4) or multidrug resistant protein-3 (MDR3) are associated with the development of ICP.[3] These genetic mutations lead to increased sensitivity to estrogen, which impairs the sulfation and transportation of bile acids. Estrogens also decrease membrane permeability and bile acid uptake by the liver. The maternal to fetal transfer of bile acids across the placenta becomes impaired, leading to potentially toxic bile acid levels in the fetus.[4] The elevation in bile acid levels is also thought

Table 8.1: Jaundice in pregnancy—causes unique to pregnancy

	ICP	*AFLP*	*PE/E*	*HELLP*	*HG*
Incidence	<10% multifetal gestations	1/13,000; primiparous, multifetal gestations	5% multiparous, multifetal gestations	0.5%	<2% primiparous
Onset	Second/third trimester	Third trimester	Second/third trimester	Third trimester	First trimester
Clinical features	Nausea, vomiting, abdominal pain, fatigue, jaundice	Nausea, vomiting, abdominal pain, fatigue, jaundice	Hypertension, edema, proteinuria, neurological deficits (headaches, seizures, coma)	Abdominal pain, nausea, vomiting, edema, hypertension, proteinuria	Nausea, vomiting, weight loss, nutritional deficiency
Histology	Centrilobular cholestasis, no inflammation	Microvesicular fat	Periportal hemorrhage, necrosis, fibrin deposits, may see microvesicular fat	Necrosis, periportal hemorrhage, fibrin deposits	Nausea, vomiting, abdominal pain, fatigue, jaundice
Specific laboratory tests	AST, ALT <1,000 IU/L; GGT normal; bile acid levels high; PT normal; bilirubin <6 mg/dL	Platelets <100,000/mm^3; AST, ALT >300 IU/L; PT elevated; fibrinogen level low; bilirubin level increased; DIC	Uric acid level elevated	Platelets <100,000/mm^3; hemolysis; high LDH level; AST, ALT 70–6,000 IU/L; DIC	AST, ALT <1,000 IU/L; ALT > AST; low TSH
Outcome	Increased gallstones; recurs; risk for fetal distress increases	Maternal mortality <20%; fetal mortality up to 45%; test for LCHAD	Maternal mortality, 1%; prematurity and fetal death, 5–30%	Hepatic rupture, with 60% maternal mortality; fetal death, 1–30%	Benign for mother and child
Treatment	Ursodeoxycholic acid; delivery recommended at 37 weeks	Prompt delivery; liver transplantation	Beta blocker, methyldopa, magnesium sulfate; early delivery	Prompt delivery	IV fluids; thiamine pyridoxine; promethazine; FDA category C

(ICP: intrahepatic cholestasis of pregnancy; AFLP: acute fatty liver of pregnancy; HELLP: hemolysis, elevated liver enzymes and low platelets; HG: hyperemesis gravidarum; PE/E: preeclampsia/eclampsia; AST: aspartate transaminase; ALT: alanine transaminase; GGT: gamma glutamyl transferase; PT: prothrombin time; LDH: lactate dehydrogenase; DIC: disseminated intravascular coagulation; TSH: thyroid-stimulating hormone; LCHAD: long-chain L-3 hydroxyacyl-CoA dehydrogenase deficiency; FDA: Food and Drug Administration)
(*Source:* (1) Jain RK. Management of jaundice in pregnancy. Medicine Update. 2010;20:470-6.
(2) Cleveland Clinic. (2010). Liver Disease in Pregnancy (Wakim-Fleming J). [online] Available from http://www.clevelandclinicmeded.com/medicalpubs/diseasemanagement/hepatology/liver-disease-in-pregnancy/ [Accessed December 2017].)

possibly to affect myometrial contractility and to cause vasoconstriction of chorionic veins in the placenta, which may contribute to preterm deliveries and fetal distress seen in ICP.[5,6]

The classic symptom is pruritus in the second or third trimester. Jaundice occurs in approximately 10–25% of patients. Cholelithiasis and cholecystitis have been observed to occur with greater frequency with ICP.[7] Total bile acid levels are elevated up to 10–25-fold. Aspartate transaminase (AST) and alanine transaminase (ALT) levels rarely exceed two times the upper limits of normal, but may approach 10–20-fold elevations in rare cases. Bilirubin levels may be elevated, but are usually less than 6 mg/dL. Serum alkaline phosphatize levels may also be elevated, but this is usually less helpful due to alkaline phosphatase elevations seen in pregnancy.

The treatment of choice is ursodeoxycholic acid (UDCA). Antihistamines are frequently used to alleviate pruritus, and vitamin K and other fat-soluble vitamin supplementation should also be administered. Delivery is generally advised at 37 weeks as fetal mortality increases beyond 37 weeks.

ACUTE FATTY LIVER OF PREGNANCY

Acute fatty liver of pregnancy is a rare but serious illness that occurs in the third trimester of pregnancy. With an incidence of 1 in 10,000 to 1 in 15,000 pregnancies, it has a maternal mortality rate of 18% and a fetal mortality rate of 23%.[8,9] AFLP is more commonly seen in nulliparous women and with multiple gestations.

The pathophysiology of AFLP involves defects in mitochondrial fatty acid beta-oxidation. When a heterozygous woman has a fetus that is homozygous for enzymatic mutations in fatty acid oxidation, fetal fatty acids accumulate and return to the mother's circulation. The extra load of long-chain fatty acids and subsequent triglyceride accumulation lead to hepatic fat deposition and impaired hepatic function in the mother. A deficiency in long-chain 3-hydroxyacyl-CoA dehydrogenase (LCHAD) is thought to be associated with the development of AFLP.[10]

Laboratory findings include elevations in aminotransferase levels, which may range from being mildly elevated to approaching 1,000 IU/L. Although liver biopsy may be helpful, it is not done due to the presence of coagulopathy.

Swansea criteria for diagnosis of AFLP (six or more criteria required in the absence of another cause):

- Vomiting
- Abdominal pain
- Polydipsia/polyuria
- Encephalopathy
- Elevated bilirubin >14 μmol/L
- Hypoglycemia <4 mmol/L
- Elevated urea >340 μmol/L
- Leukocytosis $>11 \times 10^6$ cells/L
- Ascites or bright liver on ultrasound scan

- Elevated transaminases (AST or ALT) >42 IU/L
- Elevated ammonia >47 μmol/L
- Renal impairment; creatinine >150 μmol/L
- Coagulopathy; prothrombin time >14 sec or activated partial thromboplastin time (APPT) >34 sec
- Microvesicular steatosis on liver biopsy.

Treatment of AFLP involves delivery of the fetus. In rare cases, patients will progress to fulminant hepatic failure with need for liver transplantation.[11] The baby has increased risk of cardiomyopathy, neuropathy, myopathy, nonketotic hypoglycemia, hepatic failure, and death is associated with fatty acid oxidation defects in newborns.

PREECLAMPSIA/ECLAMPSIA

Abnormal laboratory values include a 10–20-fold elevation in aminotransferases, elevations in alkaline phosphatase levels that exceed those normally observed in pregnancy, and bilirubin elevations of less than 5 mg/dL. Maternal mortality from preeclampsia/eclampsia is rare in developed countries, but may approach 15–20% in developing countries.[12] Likewise, the fetal mortality rate is rare, occurring in 1–2% of births. The only effective treatment for preeclampsia is delivery of the fetus and placenta.

HEMOLYSIS, ELEVATED LIVER ENZYMES AND LOW PLATELETS

The HELLP syndrome is a multisystemic disorder of pregnancy involving hemolysis, elevated liver tests, and low platelets. About 70% of cases occur antenatally, during the last trimester of pregnancy.[13] The pathogenesis of HELLP is thought to involve cytokines and segmental vasospasm with vascular endothelial damage. An association with a defect in LCHAD has also been described. Most patients present with right upper quadrant abdominal pain, nausea, vomiting, malaise, and edema with significant weight gain. Less commonly associated conditions include renal failure (with increased uric acid), diabetes insipidus, and antiphospholipid syndrome. Other late findings of HELLP include disseminated intravascular coagulation (DIC), pulmonary edema, placental abruption, and retinal detachment.

Laboratory findings include hemolysis with increased bilirubin levels (usually less than 5 mg/dL) and lactate dehydrogenase (LDH) levels greater than 600 IU/L, moderately elevated AST and ALT levels (200–700 IU/L), and thrombocytopenia (less than 100,000/mL). In early stages, prothrombin time and APPT are normal, but in later phases, DIC may be present with increased levels of fibrin degradation products and D-dimer, and thrombin-antithrombin complexes.

The reported maternal mortality from HELLP is 1%, and the perinatal mortality rate ranges from 7% to 22% and may be due to premature detachment of placenta, intrauterine asphyxia, and prematurity.[14] Other complications of HELLP syndrome include acute renal failure, adult respiratory distress syndrome, pulmonary edema, stroke, liver failure, and hepatic infarction. The only definitive treatment for HELLP syndrome is delivery.

HYPEREMESIS GRAVIDARUM

Hyperemesis gravidarum is defined as intractable nausea and vomiting during pregnancy leading to fluid and electrolyte imbalance, weight loss of 5% or greater and nutritional deficiency requiring hospital admission.[15] The incidence of HG varies from 0.3% to 2% of all live births.[16] HG often occurs between the 4th week and 10th week of gestation and usually resolves by the 20th week.

Liver involvement is seen in about 50–60% of patients with HG.[14] Most commonly seen are mild serum aminotransferases elevations, but there are reported cases of severe transaminase elevations (ALT levels 400 to over 1,000 U/L).[17] Mild hyperbilirubinemia with mild jaundice can be seen as well. A large cohort study has shown infants of HG mothers had lower birth weights.[18] Treatment of HG is primarily supportive. Patients should avoid triggers that aggravate nausea, and eat small, frequent, and low fat meals. Intravenous fluids, thiamine, and folate supplementation, and antiemetic therapy may be administered.

COMMON LIVER DISEASES AND PREGNANCY

Viral Hepatitis

Viral hepatitis frequently affects women of childbearing age, either as an acute infection or as a chronic disease. Hepatitis A does not appear to alter the normal course of pregnancy nor does pregnancy appear to influence the natural history of hepatitis A. Acute hepatitis E during the third trimester of pregnancy is a cause of fulminant hepatic failure and has a mortality rate of up to 20%.[19] The risks of intrauterine death and abortion in any trimester are greater in pregnant women with hepatitis E than they are in their uninfected counterparts. Maternal-fetal transmission of hepatitis E resulting in symptomatic neonatal hepatitis has been reported;[20] no known therapy will prevent vertical transmission of this virus.

Maternal hepatitis B virus infection does not influence the course of pregnancy nor does pregnancy alter the natural history of maternal hepatitis B. Most women of childbearing age with chronic hepatitis B are healthy virus carriers with a very low-risk of developing complications of their disease during gestation. Maternal-fetal transmission of hepatitis B virus is responsible for most cases of chronic hepatitis B worldwide. The infants of mothers with a reactive serum test for hepatitis B surface antigen should receive hepatitis B immunoglobulin at birth and also hepatitis B vaccine during the first day of life and at ages 1 month and 6 months.[21]

The risk for vertical transmission of hepatitis C (HCV) is about 5–10%. The risk of perinatal transmission of HCV is associated with the presence of HCV ribonucleic acid (RNA) in maternal blood at the time of birth and coinfection with human immunodeficiency virus (HIV).[22] Prolonged rupture of membranes (greater than 6 hours) has also been associated with an increased risk of perinatal HCV transmission; thus, it is advised that the second stage of labor be kept short in HCV-infected pregnant women.[23]

AUTOIMMUNE LIVER DISEASE

Autoimmune hepatitis is more common in women. Treated women who subsequently conceive a child should continue taking immunosuppressive medications during pregnancy. The doses of azathioprine prescribed as part of standard treatment regimens are believed not to be teratogenic.

HEMOLYTIC JAUNDICE: SICKLE CELL ANEMIA WITH PREGNANCY

Pregnancy is high-risk in sickle cell disease. Hemolytic crisis causes rapidly developing anemia with jaundice. Hepatosplenomegaly, heart failure is common. Increased incidence of maternal preeclampsia, partum hemorrhage (PPH), and infection. Increased morbidity and mortality are due to cerebrovascular accident (CVA), pulmonary infarction, congestive heart failure (CHF), embolism, etc. There is increased risk of abortion, prematurity, intrauterine growth restriction (IUGR), fetal loss, and perinatal mortality.

CHOLELITHIASIS

Pregnancy alters bile composition and gallbladder emptying slows in the second trimester increasing the risk of gallstones. Choledocholithiasis accounts for approximately 7% of patients with jaundice in pregnancy but jaundice occurs in only 5% of cholelithiasis. There is increased risk of morbidity and mortality for both mother and fetus because of cholangitis and pancreatitis. Treatment involves laparoscopic cholecystectomy. Uncomplicated cholecystectomy is safer in first and second trimesters with fetal loss about 5%, but with common bile duct exploration and if with pancreatitis then 15% maternal and 60% fetal mortality is seen.

CONCLUSION

Jaundice in pregnancy should be evaluated thoroughly with proper history, clinical examination, and laboratory investigation to identify the underlying cause. Proper management may improve maternal and fetal outcome.

REFERENCES

1. Reyes H. Review: intrahepatic cholestasis. A puzzling disorder of pregnancy. J Gastroenterol Hepatol. 1997;12:211-6.

2. Tan LK. Obstetric cholestasis: current opinions and management. Ann Acad Med Singapore. 2003;32:294-8.
3. Jacquemin E, Cresteil D, Manouvrier S, et al. Heterozygous non-sense mutation of the MDR3 gene in familial intrahepatic cholestasis of pregnancy. Lancet. 1999;353:210-1.
4. Rodrigues CM, Marin JJ, Brites D. Bile acid patterns in meconium are influenced by cholestasis of pregnancy and not altered by ursodeoxycholic acid treatment. Gut. 1999;45:446-52.
5. Sepulveda WH, Gonzalez C, Cruz MA, et al. Vasoconstrictive effect of bile acids on isolated human placental chorionic veins. Eur J Obstet Gynecol Reprod Biol. 1991;42:211-5.
6. Germain AM, Kato S, Carvajal JA, et al. Bile acids increase response and expression of human myometrial oxytocin receptor. Am J Obstet Gynecol. 2003;189:577-82.
7. Ropponen A, Sund R, Riikonen S, et al. Intrahepatic cholestasis of pregnancy as an indicator of liver and biliary diseases: a population-based study. Hepatology. 2006;43:723-8.
8. Knox TA, Olans LB. Liver disease in pregnancy. N Engl J Med. 1996;335:569-76.
9. Castro MA, Fassett MJ, Reynolds TB, et al. Reversible peripartum liver failure: a new perspective on the diagnosis, treatment, and cause of acute fatty liver of pregnancy, based on 28 consecutive cases. Am J Obstet Gynecol. 1999;181:389-95.
10. Ibdah JA. Acute fatty liver of pregnancy: an update on pathogenesis and clinical implications. World J Gastroenterol. 2006;12:7397-404.
11. Ockner SA, Brunt EM, Cohn SM, et al. Fulminant hepatic failure caused by acute fatty liver of pregnancy treatedby orthotopic liver transplantation. Hepatology. 1990;11:59-64.
12. Sibai B, Dekker G, Kupferminc M. Pre-eclampsia. Lancet. 2005;365:785-99.
13. Sibai BM, Ramadan MK, Usta I, et al. Maternal morbidity and mortality in 442 pregnancies with hemolysis, elevated liver enzymes, and low platelets (HELLP syndrome). Am J Obstet Gynecol. 1993;169:1000-6.
14. Hepburn IS, Schade RR. Pregnancy-associated liver disorders. Dig Dis Sci. 2008;53:2334-58.
15. Fairweather DV. Nausea and vomiting in pregnancy. Am J Obstet Gynecol. 1968;102:135-75.
16. Kallen B. Hyperemesis during pregnancy and delivery outcome: a registry study. Eur J Obstet Gynecol Reprod Biol. 1987;26:291-302.
17. Conchillo JM, Pijnenborg JM, Peeters P, et al. Liver enzyme elevation induced by hyperemesis gravidarum: aetiology, diagnosis and treatment. Neth J Med. 2002;60:374-8.
18. Bailit JL. Hyperemesis gravidarium: Epidemiologic findings from a large cohort. Am J Obstet Gynecol. 2005;193:811-4.
19. Khuroo MS, Teli MR, Skidmore S, et al. Incidence and severity of viral hepatitis in pregnancy. Am J Med. 1981;70:252-5.
20. Rab MA, Bile MK, Mubarik MM, et al. Water-borne hepatitis E virus epidemic in Islamabad, Pakistan: A common source outbreak traced to the malfunction of a modern water treatment plant. Am J Trop Med Hyg. 1997;57:151-7.
21. American Academy of Pediatrics Committee on Infectious Diseases: Universal hepatitis B immunization. Pediatrics. 1992;89:795-800.
22. Conte D, Fraquelli M, Prati D, et al. Prevalence and clinical course of chronic hepatitis C virus (HCV) infection and rate of HCV vertical transmission in a cohort of 15,250 pregnant women. Hepatology. 2000;31:751-5.
23. Mast EE, Hwang LY, Seto DS, et al. Risk factors for perinatal transmission of hepatitis C virus (HCV) and the natural history of HCV infection acquired in infancy. J Infect Dis. 2005;192:1880-9.

Chapter 10

Management of Monochorionic Twins

Lucy Das

INTRODUCTION

The increase in multiple births during the past 30 years has been well documented. Making multiple gestations one of the most common high-risk conditions encountered by obstetricians. The increase in multiples is primarily due to assisted reproduction technology but childbearing at elderly age is also a risk factor.

Twin birth rates have raised 70% from 1980 to 2004. But in 2004, the rate is almost stable at 32.1/1000. This is mainly due to refreshments of assisted reproduction technologies and limitations of number of embryo transfer in in vitro fertilization (IVF).

ZYGOSITY AND CHRONICITY

Twins can be monozygotic (Mz) or dizygotic (DZ). Zygotic refers to the genetic makeup of the twin pregnancy and chronicity indicates the pregnancy's placental composition. Chronicity is determined by the mechanism of twining and in Mz twins by the timing of embryo division. Early determination of chronicity is vital because it is a major factor in determining obstetrical risks management and outcome.

Dizygotic twins result from the fertilization of two different ova and two separate sperms. Dichorionic and diamniotic placentation occurs in DZ twin because each blastocyst develops its own placenta. Mz twin pregnancy in created by the fertilization of one ova and one sperm and then subsequent spontaneous cleavage of the fertilized ovum. Thus, the type of placentations that develops is determined by the timing of the cleavage.

- *Cleavage within 3 days:* Dichorionic and diamniotic
- *Cleavage at 4–7 days:* Monochorionic and diamniotic
- *Cleavage at 8–12 days:*- Monochorionic and monoamniotic
- *Cleavage after 13 days:* Conjoint twin.

Among natural conception DZ twins arise in about 1.1–1.5 % of pregnancies whereas Mz twins occur in 1 in 250 pregnancies. MZ twining rates are constant across all variables with the exception of assisted reproduction. Rate of MZ twining may be more than 10-folds higher in pregnancies by assisted reproductive technology (ART) than spontaneous conception. It may be due to injury to Zona pellucida causing iatrogenic zygote splitting.

DIAGNOSIS OF MULTIPLE GESTATION

First Trimester

Using vaginal ultrasound separate gestational sac with individual yolk sac can be identified as early as 5 weeks of pregnancy and cardiac activity can be seen by 6 weeks.

Accurate determinations of chorionicity is essential in counseling patients on obstetrics and neonatal risks because chronicity is a major determinant of pregnancy outcome and it is easily detectable at first trimester by ultrasonography (USG). Chronicity can be diagnosed by USG between 6–10 weeks of pregnancy by counting the number of gestational sacs and evaluating the thickness of dividing membrane.

Two separate gestational sac each containing a fetus and thick dividing membrane suggest a dichorionic diamniotic pregnancy, whereas one gestational sac with a thin dividing membrane with two fetuses suggest a monochorionic pregnancy.

After 9 weeks the dividing membrane becomes progressively thinner in monochorionic twin but in dichorionic twin they remain thicker and easy to identify.

Second Trimester

At 12–14 weeks "Twin peak sign" or lambda sign will help to differentiate between dichorionic and monochorionic pregnancy. On examining the base of the intertwin membrane twin peak sign can be seen. It is a triangular projection of tissue identified beyond the chorionic surface of placenta. This sign is seen in dichorionic twin not in monochorionic twin.

In second trimester, chorionicity of a fetus can be accessed by determining the number of placentas, the sex of each fetus and the membrane that divide the sacs. This is helpful having 91.7% sensitivity and 97.3% specificity for diagnosis of monochorionicity as studied by Scardo and associates in 2009.[1]

TYPES OF MONOCHORIONIC TWIN

Out of all Monochorionic Twins

- Monochorionic diamniotic—70–75%
- Monochorionic monoamniotic—20%
- Conjoint twins—5%.

Monochorionic Diamniotic Twin

It is the most commonly occurred monochorionic twin.

MONOCHORIONIC MONOAMNIOTIC

They are relatively rare occurring about 1 in 12,500 births. They are associated with high prenatal mortality (approximately 50%). Most common cause of death is umbilical cord entanglement.

Two-thirds of the fetal death involves both fetuses and one-third-one of the fetus.

Monoamniotic twins occur frequently following assisted reproduction techniques that involve manipulation of the Zona Pellucidum.

CONJOINT TWIN

Incidence is 1 in every 200 Mz twin or 1 in 50,000 births. This occurs when cleavage takes place after 13th day of conception.

Classification according to sight of union:
- Thoracophagus—joint at chest (19%)
- Omphalophagus—Joint at anterior abdominal wall (18%)
- Ischiophagus—Joint at Ischium (11%)
- Carniopagus— Joint at Head (11%).

Ultrasonography findings:
- Twins face each other
- Heads are at same level and place
- The thoracic cages are in unusual proximity
- Both fetal head are hyperextended
- No change in relative position.

The outcome of conjoint twin in poor as 40% will be still born and 35% will die within 1 day or delivery.

Complications of Monochorionic Twins

- Vanishing twins and intrauterine fetal death: At first trimester pregnancy one fetus may lose cardiac activity and the pregnancies can be continued with the other fetus. Except little vaginal bleeding usually no risk occurs.
- Intrauterine fetal death (IUFD):Fetal death of one twin can occur in second or third trimester in about 2.5–6.8% twin pregnancy. Severe sequelae can occur in the surviving twin like multiorgan damage or preterm labor. Fetal death may be due to genetic and anatomic anomalies, abruption, placental insufficiency, cord abnormalities, gestational diabetes mellitus (GDM), pregnancy-induced hypertension (PIH), cord entanglement, etc.
- *Twin-twin transfusion syndrome (TTTS):* It is typical to monochorionic diamniotic twins and seen in 15% monochorionic gestation. It is characterized by an imbalance of fetal blood flow through communicating

vessels across common placenta leading to under perfusion of donor twin and over perfusion of recipient twin.

- *Acardiac Twin:* This malformation occurs only in monochorionic twin. Over all morbidity is 60–70% in second trimester and almost 100% in third trimester.
- Congenital anomaly
- *Umbilical cord problems (mostly seen in monochorionic and monoamniotic twin):*
  - Cord entanglement
  - Velamentous insertion of cord
- Cerebral palsy.

Twin-to-twin Transfusion

Diagnostic Criteria of Twin-to-twin to Transfusion during Pregnancy

- Only one placenta is seen by USG
- Twins are of same sex
- There is thin membrane between the two twins (diamniotic placentation)
- There is a 20% or more discordancy in estimated fetal weight between the twins
- There is a significant discrepancy in the amniotic fluid volume surrounding each twins
- Fetal hydrops is present in one or both twins
- The umbilical cords are of different size.

Feature of Donor Twin

- Retarded growth
- Hydrops fetalis
- High-output heart failure
- Poor growth
- Oliguria
- Anemia
- Hyperproteinemia.

Features of Recipient Twin

Features occur due to increase in cardiac volume.

- Cardiomegaly
- Cardiac congestive failure (CCF)
- Respiratory defects
- Intrauterine fetal death
- Hyperbilirubinemia.

Neonatal Diagnosis of Twin–twin Transfusion Syndrome

- Difference in hemoglobin equal to or larger than 5 g/dL
- Difference in birthweight greater than 20%.

Quintero's classification of severity of TTT's:

- *Stage 1:* Oligopoly sequence and bladder seen in the donor twin
- *Stage 2:* Oligopoly sequence, donor bladder not seen, normal Doppler studies
- *Stage 3:* Oligopoly sequence, donor bladder not seen Doppler with at least one of the following alterations:
  - Absent or reversed diastolic flow in the umbilical artery in the donor twins
  - Reverse flow in the ductus venosus of the donor twin
  - Pulsatile flow in the umbilical vein of the recipient twin.
- *Stage 4:* Fetal hydrops in any of the twins
- *Stage 5:* Death of one or both twins.

Management

- Serial amnioreduction
- Laser ablation of vascular anastomosis between the twin
- Amniotic septostomy (perforation of intertwin amniotic membrane)
- Selective feticide.

Acardiac Twin

Incidence—1 in 35,000 births. In this case, one twin has no cardiac structures or placental circulation and the blood supply come from the healthy twin by means of arterio-arterial (AA) anastomosis. Blood of donor twin enter the acardiac twin via umbilical artery and iliac vessels. The arterial system of the acardiac twin is perfused in reverse with deoxygenated blood from the normal twin (twin reversed arterial perfusion or TRAP).

Management

- Serial amniocentesis
- Selective removal of acardiac twin
- Insertion of a thrombogenic coil in the umbilical artery of the acardiac twin
- Interruption of the AA anastomosis between the donor and acardiac twin.

MATERNAL RISK IN MULTIPLE PREGNANCY

All the obstetrics complications with exception of macrosomia are elevated with multiple gestations and are likely to have more severe manifestation of those conditions.

Antenatal and Postnatal Complications

The complications of antenatal and postnatal are given in the Table 9.1.

Table 9.1: Complications of antenatal and postnatal.

	Twin (%)	*Single ton (%)*
Hypertension	5.1	1.7
Threatened abortion	26.5	18.6
Anemia	27.5	16.2
Abruption	1.9	0.5
GHTN	23.8	17.8
PET	11.5	3.4
Eclampsia	0.2	0.1
MROP	6.7	2.5
PPH	3.1	0.9
Postpartum thromboembolism	0.6	0.2

(GHTN: gestational hypertension; PET: pre-eclamptic toxemia; PPH: postpartum hemorrhage; MROP: manual removal of placental tissue)

Perinatal Morbidity and Mortality

Babies delivered from multiple gestations have higher rates of low birth weight, preterm birth, infant deaths, and fetal anomalies.

A 2009 population-based study found that rate of congenital anomalies were 1.7 times more in twins compared to single ton pregnancy and more so in Mz twins.[2]

Management of Monochorionic Twin

- *Antepartum:*
  - Prevention of preterm births
  - Rest
  - Prophylactic tocolysis
  - Betamethasone injection two doses
  - Home uterine activity monitoring
  - Infection surveillance
  - Testing fetal fibronectin
  - Cervical length assessment by USG
  - Cervical cerclage.
- *Fetal growth assessment:*
  - To be done by USG every 2 weeks after 20 weeks
  - Discordant growth—15–29% pregnancies are affected
  - Screening for chromosomal abnormalities—nuchal translucency (NT) scan at 11–13 weeks and quadruples test in second trimester
  - Biophysical profile monitoring
  - Fetal lung maturation.

Management in Labor

- *Timing of delivery*:
  - Uncomplicated monochromic diamniotic twin should be delivered at 36 weeks because beyond that the risk of fetal demise is greater
  - In monochorionic monoamniotic pregnancy should be delivered by caesarean at 32 weeks because chance of cord entanglement and subsequent fetal death prevails more after this.
- *Routine of delivery:*
  - According to the presentation of 1st baby and birth weight, decision may be taken for vaginal delivery or lower segment cesarian section (LSCS) in [monochorionic-diamniotic (Mo–Di)] twin
  - Lower segment cesarian section pregnant in (Mo–Mo) twin
  - In conjoint twin delivery usually done by cesarean section unless it is very early pregnancy and vaginal expulsion of both is possible.

REFERENCES

1. Scardo JA, Ellings JM, Newyork RB. Prospective determination of chorionicity, amniocity and zygosity in twin gestations. AM J Obstate Gynecol. 1995;173(5):1376-80.
2. American College of Obstetricians and Gynecologists (ACOG). Special problems of multiple Gestations, Educational Bulletin No.253. Washington, DC: ACOG; 1998.
3. Baldwin VJ, Wittmen BK. Pathology of intragestational intervention in twin–twin transfusion syndrome. Pediatr Pathol. 1990;10(1-2):79-93.
4. D'Alton ME, Dudely DK. The ultrasonographic prediction of chorionicity in twin gestation. Am J Obstet Gynecol. 1989;160(3):557-61.
5. Goldenberg RL, Iams JD, Miodovnik M, et al. The preterm prediction study: Risk factors in twin gestation. Am J Obstet Gynecol. 1996:175(4 pt 1):1047-53.
6. Lopriore E, Middeldorp JM, Sueters M, et al. Long-term neurodevelopmental outcome in twin- twin transfusion syndrome treated with fetoscopic laser surgery. Am J Obstate Gynacol. 2007;196(3):231.e l-4.
7. Quintero RA, Morales WJ, Allen MH, et al. Staging of twin–twin transfusion syndrome. J Perinatol. 1999;19(8 pt 1):550-5.
8. Winn HN, Gabrielli S, Reece EA, et al. Ultrasonographic criteria for the prenatal diagnosis of placental chorionicity in twin gestations. AM J Obstate gynacol. 1989;161(6 Pt l):1540-2.

Chapter 11

Unexplained Fetal Death

Chaitali Dutta

ABSTRACT

The loss of a fetus at any stage is distressing, and when unexplained, it is an unexpected, devastating complication. The WHO defines fetal death as "death prior to complete expulsion or extraction from the mother, regardless of the duration of pregnancy." This is considered unexplained when known etiologies are not documented after thorough autopsy and histopathological examination. According to data published by the WHO in 2015 there were 2.6 million stillbirths globally, with more than 7,178 deaths a day. Although half of all stillbirths occur during the intrapartum period, the rest may be attributed to intrauterine fetal demise. Of these cases, 25–60% remain unexplained, and thus this area continues to be a major challenge in obstetrics.

PRESENTATION AND DIAGNOSIS

In most patients, the only symptom is decreased fetal movement. Although on auscultation inability to obtain fetal heart tones is suspicious, ideally death must be confirmed by real-time ultrasound. A second opinion should be obtained whenever practically possible. The mother should be prepared for the possibility of passive fetal movement and if she reports such, a repeat scan should be offered. Certain secondary features may also be seen, e.g. collapse of the fetal skull with overlapping bones, hydrops, maceration and even intrafetal gas (within the heart, blood vessels and joints). Once diagnosed, management needs to be directed both towards ascertaining the cause of death, and terminating the pregnancy with minimal risk to the mother.

ASCERTAINING THE CAUSE OF FETAL DEATH

Attempting to determine the cause of fetal death remains important because it may influence estimates of recurrence, future preconception counseling, pregnancy management, prenatal diagnostic procedures and neonatal management. Another important purpose of investigation is to assess present maternal wellbeing and ensure prompt management of any potentially life-threatening maternal disease.

When identifiable, fetal death can be attributable to maternal, fetal or placental pathologies. The major causes of fetal loss in each of the trimesters can be summarized as follows:

- *First trimester:* genetic abnormalities
- *Second trimester:* fetal infection and placental thrombosis
- *Third trimester:* cord accident and placental thrombosis.

Among the maternal causes are hypertension, diabetes, systemic lupus erythematosus, antiphospholipid syndrome, inherited thrombophilias, infection, hemoglobinopathy, Rh disease, uterine rupture and prolonged pregnancy. Fetal factors include multiple gestations, intrauterine growth restriction, congenital abnormality, genetic abnormality, infection (parvovirus B19, CMV, *Listeria*) and hydrops. Placental changes related to hypercoagulability are detected in many cases of intrauterine fetal death (IUFD). These changes include infarcts, thrombosis, and obliteration of blood vessels. Other placental causes include abruption, premature rupture of membranes, vasa previa, fetomaternal hemorrhage and cord accidents. Cord accidents may be due to coiling and an important distinction should be made between the types of coiling (type A or B) to assess the degree of risk. Type A encirclement can undo itself, as the placental insertion end crosses over the umbilical insertion end. On the other hand, in type B coil the placental end crosses under the umbilical end, and therefore becomes locked. These type B encirclements are the ones that increase fetal risk. Again, marginal insertions appear more prone to vessel rupture or compression while velamentous cord insertions are susceptible to folding and torsion of umbilical vessels. Trophoblast inclusions, which are abnormal infoldings of the villus trophoblast bilayer, have been proposed as a marker of genetically abnormal gestations and could be clinically useful when a karyotype could not be performed.

A number of risk factors have also been associated with fetal death. The incidence of fetal death varies according to maternal race as evidenced in the United States where the rate is higher in black compared to white women. Maternal obesity and smoking are considered the top modifiable factors. Along with these, advanced maternal age (>35 years), single marital status, low education, history of fetal demise, maternal infertility and paternal age have been implicated.

Obesity is known to be associated with disturbances in the endocrine system and lipid metabolism. Hyperlipidemia, through a reduction in prostacycline secretion and elevation of thromboxane production, may increase the risk of placental thrombosis and decrease placental perfusion. Associated insulin resistance, where fibrinolytic activity is known to be decreased, leads to impaired placental blood flow which may explain the increased risk of stillbirth found in obese women.

The other known culprit, prenatal smoke exposure enables carbon monoxide to cross placenta and bind to hemoglobin causing fetal hypoxia by increased blood levels of carboxyhemoglobin. This probably interferes with fetal immune system predisposing to infections, as well as causing damage to developing organs. Alterations (hypoplasia to agenesis) of arcuate nucleus is detectable and mutation of the gene *En-2* on chromosome 7 is thought to be involved as a consequence of smoke exposure.

THEORIES TO EXPLAIN THE UNEXPLAINED

Extensive studies have been conducted in an attempt to fathom the unknown causes of fetal demise.

Increased Anti-angiogenic Factors

Intrauterine growth restriction has been proposed to be responsible for majority of *unexplained* fetal death cases. Fetal growth and placental development require a balance between angiogenic and anti-angiogenic processes. The main regulator for angiogenesis is vascular endothelial growth factor (VEGF)—signaling system. The presence of increased concentrations of anti-angiogenic factors in amniotic fluid may help explain the pathophysiology in such cases. Decreased concentration of placental growth factor (PlGF) and elevated concentrations of anti-angiogenic molecules, such as soluble vascular endothelial growth factor receptor-1 (sVEGFR-1) and soluble endoglin (sEng) have also been identified in the maternal circulation in these patients.

Dysregulated Maternal Immune Response

The complement system normally plays a central role in innate immunity. Pregnancy is characterized by expression of paternal alloantigens in fetal tissue that can elicit both a humoral and a cellular immune response yet most pregnancies are successful, suggesting that there is tolerance to these alloantigens. Complement activation is part of a compensatory state of the innate immune response during pregnancy, when the adaptive immune response is suppressed presumably to allow tolerance of the fetal semi-allograft. Some pregnancy losses have been attributed to a dysregulated maternal immune response against fetal antigens. Studies have demonstrated that pregnant women with unexplained fetal death have a higher median plasma C5a concentration. It is possible that a subclinical maternal and/or fetal infection may account for the high maternal plasma concentration of C5a among cases with unexplained intrauterine death.

Sudden Intrauterine Unexplained Death Syndrome (SIUDS)

Sudden infant death syndrome (SIDS) is considered an important cause of mortality during the first year of life and has been attributed to long-QT syndrome (LQTS). This is characterized by an abnormality in cardiac repolarization that leads to prolongation of the QT interval and T wave changes. Direct and indirect evidence that some deaths from SIUDS are caused by long QT syndrome (LQTS) has been published. This has made it possible to establish a link between SIDS and unexplained fetal death and opened up the possibility to perform in-utero pharmacologic therapy.

Biological Signature of Maternal Anti-fetal Rejection

Chronic chorioamnionitis is a major placental lesion in clinically unexplained preterm fetal death. It is defined as amniotrophic infiltration of maternal T cells into the chorioamniotic membranes and may be considered a histological manifestation of maternal anti-fetal cellular rejection occurring in the chorioamniotic membranes. The fetus is a semi-allogeneic graft to the mother, and its survival is a key parameter of successful reproduction. Fetal death therefore might be analogous to the failure of graft survival in organ transplantation. Patients with chronic chorioamnionitis have a history of spontaneous abortion, fetal death or preterm birth. These three conditions could actually be different manifestations of a common pathophysiology: maternal anti-fetal rejection.

RECOMMENDED TESTS

In order to determine, the cause of fetal demise numerous investigations including blood culture, midstream urine, vaginal swab, serology, blood sugar, thyroid function, thrombophilia screen (if abnormal, repeat at 6 weeks), antiphospholipid screen (repeated if abnormal), anti-Ro and anti-La antibodies, factor V leiden, prothrombin mutation and parental karyotype are advised.

POSTMORTEM EXAMINATION

- Fetal autopsy and placental evaluation
- Tissue samples should be placed in sterile medium from the cytogenetics laboratory or sterile saline solution and kept at room temperature. When the parents refuse a complete autopsy, postmortem MRI can also be done.

TERMINATION OF PREGNANCY

Although labor usually ensues spontaneously in fetal demise, fibrinogen levels may drop, leading to coagulopathy, when a dead fetus has been in utero for 3–4 weeks. Nowadays, this is rarely a problem because of early recognition and management. Vaginal birth is the recommended mode of delivery for most women, but cesarean birth will need to be considered with some. Sometimes induction after the death of a twin may be delayed to allow the viable twin to mature and these women should be advised DIC twice weekly. Women should be advised immediate delivery if there is sepsis, preeclampsia, placental abruption or membrane rupture.

Induction may be accomplished with preinduction cervical ripening followed by intravenous oxytocin. Mifepristone 200 mg orally followed by misoprostol orally or vaginally appears to be efficacious and where mifepristone is unavailable, misoprostol alone is also highly effective. Prostaglandin E2 (PGE2) suppositories can also be administered until labor is induced. Certain colleges recommend that misoprostol not be used for cervical ripening or labor induction in women with prior uterine incisions. Here mechanical ripening can be performed with a Foley catheter, and induction can be continued with oxytocin but it should be remembered that mechanical methods of induction might increase the risk of ascending infection in the presence of IUFD. Mifepristone can be used alone to increase the chance of labor significantly within 72 hours (avoiding the use of prostaglandin). Pain management in patients undergoing induction of labor for fetal demise is an important part of patient care. Dopamine agonists successfully suppress lactation and cabergoline is superior to bromocriptine, but they should not be given to women with hypertension or pre-eclampsia as they can increase blood pressure and have been associated with intracerebral hemorrhage.

PREGNANCY FOLLOWING UNEXPLAINED STILLBIRTH

Women with a previous unexplained IUFD should be recommended screening for gestational diabetes. For women in whom a normally formed stillborn baby had evidence of being small for gestational age, serial assessment of growth by ultrasound biometry should be recommended in subsequent pregnancies.

Chapter 12

Preterm Premature Rupture of Membranes—An Enigma

Sukumar Barik

INTRODUCTION

Premature rupture of membranes (PROM) is the rupture of membranes before the onset of labor. Membrane rupture before labor and before 37 weeks of gestation is referred to as preterm premature rupture of membranes (PPROM). PPROM is far more difficult to manage than PROM at term. The best possible approach to clinical assessment and treatment of women with term and PPROM remains controversial. A number of issues need to be considered in formulating a plan of management. Prematurity is the most important risk to the fetus, while infection and its complications are the principal maternal risks. The management of PPROM depends on the balance between the risks for fetal and neonatal complications with immediate delivery versus the risks and benefits of conservative treatment. The neonatal risks are primarily gestational-age-related. Therefore, the initial steps include confirmation of membrane rupture in addition to assessment of estimated gestational age, duration of membrane rupture, exclusion of maternal infection or abruption and assessment of fetal well being. Expectant management and immediate delivery are potential options in these patients, and each has its own advantages and disadvantages. With appropriate care, the maternal risks of expectant management are generally expected to be minimal and a clear neonatal advantage exists by reducing risks of prematurity.

EXPECTANT MANAGEMENT—USUAL OUTCOME

- At term, PROM complicates approximately 8% of pregnancies and is generally followed by the prompt onset of spontaneous labor and delivery.
- Regardless of obstetric management or clinical presentation, birth within 1 week of membrane rupture occurs in at least one half of patients with preterm PROM.

- The earlier the PROM occurs, the greater is the latency period
- Spontaneous sealing of the membranes does occur occasionally (<10% of all the cases), mostly after PPROM that has occurred subsequent to amniocentesis; however, this is very uncommon.

Diagnosis

- Most cases of PROM can be diagnosed on the basis of the patient's history and physical examination
- A sterile speculum examination demonstrating pooling of fluid in the posterior vaginal fornix is done in selected cases. Sterile speculum examination provides an opportunity to inspect for cervicitis and umbilical cord prolapse or fetal prolapse, assess cervical dilatation and effacement, and obtain cultures as appropriate
- Digital cervical examinations increase the risk of infection and add little information to that available with speculum examination
- Digital examinations generally should be avoided unless the patient appears to be inactive labor or delivery seems imminent
- A Nitrazine paper test or fern test has no significant value in modern practice
- Ultrasound examination is helpful in some cases to find reduced liquor
- In addition, ultrasonography provides information about the fetal condition and the status of the cervix
- Fetal fibronectin test has a limitation of poor predictive value because of high false positive rate. Therefore despite high (98–99%) negative predictive value, its use is not recommended.

EXPECTANT MANAGEMENT OF PRETERM PROM

- Hospital admission with periodic assessment for infection, abruptio placentae, umbilical cord compression, fetal well-being, and labor
- The criteria for the diagnosis of clinical chorioamnionitis include maternal pyrexia, tachycardia, leukocytosis, uterine tenderness, offensive vaginal discharge and fetal tachycardia
- Serial monitoring of leukocyte counts and other markers of inflammation have not been proved to be useful and are nonspecific when there is no clinical evidence of infection
- There is no consensus on the optimal frequency of assessment, but an acceptable strategy would include periodic ultrasonographic monitoring of fetal growth and periodic fetal heart rate monitoring
- Weekly high vaginal swab need not be performed
- CTG is useful and indeed fetal tachycardia is used in the definition of clinical chorioamnionitis
- Biophysical profile score and Doppler velocimetry can be carried out, but these tests are of limited value in predicting fetal infection.

Antibiotics use in PPROM

- Offer women with oral erythromycin 250 mg 4 times a day for a maximum of 10 days or until the woman is in established labor (whichever is sooner)
- For women who cannot tolerate erythromycin or in whom use of erythromycin is contraindicated, consider oral penicillin for a maximum of 10 days or until the woman is in established labor (whichever is sooner)
- Do not offer women with co-amoxiclav as prophylaxis for intrauterine infection.

Tocolytics in PPROM

- The use of tocolysis in the setting of PPROM is controversial and practice patterns among specialists vary widely
- Prophylactic tocolysis may be associated with a prolongation of pregnancy and an increased risk of chorioamnionitis without significant maternal or neonatal benefit
- Available data do not support the routine use of either prophylactic or therapeutic tocolysis after PPROM.

Corticosteroids in PPROM

- Use of a course of corticosteroid reduces neonatal mortality, respiratory distress syndrome, intraventricular hemorrhage, and necrotizing enterocolitis
- Antenatal steroid therapy does not increase the risks of neonatal or maternal infection irrespective of gestational age
- Offer maternal corticosteroids to women between 26+0 and 33+6 weeks of pregnancy that are in suspected, or diagnosed have PPROM
- Consider maternal corticosteroids for women between 34+0 and 35+6 weeks of pregnancy who a have PPROM.

Time to Deliver

Prior to 32 weeks

- The evidence suggests expectant management with antibiotics and steroids in absence of any complication (infection, abruption, active labor or non-reassuring fetal heart)
- However, long-term outcome of these preterm infants are a real concern.

Between 32–34 weeks

- Some group recommends aggressive approach to delivery since the risk of infection increases with expectancy
- The management remains controversial until the long-term outcome of the infants delivered electively during this gestational age is available.

Greater than or in 34 weeks

Most recommended delivery since little benefit is likely to accrue following expectant management.

TWIN PREGNANCIES WITH PPROM

- Currently, there is a paucity of robust data. Therefore recommendations for management of such women are extrapolated from studies in singletons
- Monochorionic twins need special considerations
- During expectancy administration of course, antenatal steroids and antibiotics seem reasonable
- However, management should better be individualized.

FURTHER READING

1. Preterm labour and birth. NICE guideline 2015 [online]. Available from: www.nice.org.uk/guidance/ng25
2. Practice Bulletin No. 172: Premature Rupture of Membranes. Obstet Gynecol. 2016;128(4):e165-77.

Chapter 13

Screening and Management of Gestational Diabetes

Sujata Misra

INTRODUCTION

Pregnancy induces progressive changes in maternal carbohydrate metabolism. As pregnancy advances insulin resistance and diabetogenic stress due to placental hormones necessitate compensatory increase in insulin secretion. When this compensation is inadequate gestational diabetes develops which is defined as carbohydrate intolerance with onset or recognition during pregnancy. Women diagnosed to have gestational diabetes mellitus (GDM) are at increased risk of future diabetes predominantly type 2 DM as are their children. Thus, GDM offers an important opportunity for the development, testing and implementation of clinical strategies for diabetes prevention.

SCREENING AND DIAGNOSIS

A number of screening procedures and diagnostic criteria [American Diabetes Association (ADA), World Health Organization (WHO), Canadian Diabetes Association (CDA), National Diabetes Data Group (NDDG) and Australasian criteria] are being followed in the same as well as in different countries.

American Diabetes Association Procedure

American Diabetes Association recommends two step procedures. *Step 1:* A 50 g glucose challenge test (GCT) is used for screening without regard to the time of last meal or time of the day. *Step 2:* If 1 hour GCT value is more than 140 mg/dL, 100 g oral glucose tolerance test (OGTT) is recommended and plasma glucose is estimated at 0, 1, 2 and 3 hours. Gestational diabetes mellitus is diagnosed (Carpenter and Coustan criteria) if any 2 values meet or exceed FPG >95 mg/dL, 1 hour PG >180 mg/dL, 2 hour PG >155 mg/dL and 3 hour PG >140 mg/dL. The drawback of these criteria is that, the glycemic cut off was originally validated against the future risk of these women developing diabetes and not on the fetal outcome. Further,

1. The number of blood samples drawn are many—(a) for screening and (b) for subsequent 3-hour OGTT to confirm the diagnosis (4 blood samples).
2. They have to visit the antenatal clinic on two occasions—(a) for screening and (b) again for diagnostic procedure.

WHO Procedure

World Health Organization recommends using a 2 hour 75 g OGTT with a threshold plasma glucose concentration of greater than 140 mg/dL at 2 hours, similar to that of IGT (>140 and <199 mg/dL), outside pregnancy. When a glucose tolerance test is administered to a nonpregnant individual, it is standard to use the 75-g, 2-hour OGTT (Table 1). Using a different glucose challenge in pregnant versus nonpregnant persons leads to confusion in the laboratory and may result in errors in applying the proper diagnostic criteria.

A Single Test Procedure to Diagnose Gestational Diabetes Mellitus in the Community

It is important to have a test that detects the glucose intolerance without the woman necessarily undergoing a test in the fasting state and it is preferable to perform the diagnostic test at the first visit itself (Box 1).

Performing this test procedure in the nonfasting state is rational, as glucose concentrations are affected little by the time since the last meal in a normal glucose tolerant woman, whereas it will, in a woman with gestational diabetes. This single step procedure serves both as screening and diagnostic test for GDM, is simple, economical and feasible.

Table 1: With 75 g oral glucose tolerance test (OGTT) (World Health Organization criteria)

Plasma Glucose	*In Pregnancy*	*Outside Pregnancy*
2 hour ≥200 mg/dL	Diabetes	Diabetes
2 hour ≥140 mg/dL and ≤199 mg/dL	GDM	IGT
2 hour ≥120 mg/dL and ≤139 mg/dL	GGI	—
2 hour <120 mg/dL	Normal	Normal

Box 1: Test procedure to diagnose gestational diabetes mellitus.

In the antenatal clinic, a pregnant woman after undergoing preliminary clinical examination, has to be given a 75 g oral glucose load*, without regard to the time of the last meal. A venous blood sample is collected at 2 hours for estimating plasma glucose by the GOD-POD method. GDM is diagnosed if 2 hour plasma glucose is ≥140 mg/dL.

*If 75 g glucose packet is not available, remove 5 level teaspoons (not heaped) of glucose from a 100 g packet which is freely available. In hospitals where glucose is supplied in bulk, a cup or container of 75 g may be used.

Advantages:
- The pregnant women need not be fasting.
- Causes least disturbance in a pregnant woman's routine activities.
- Serves as both screening and diagnostic procedure.

Gestational Weeks at which Screening is Recommended

Insulin is detectable in the fetal pancreas as early as 9 weeks after conception. By following the usual recommendation for screening between 24 weeks and 28 weeks of gestation, the chance of detecting unrecognized type 2 diabetes before pregnancy (pre-GDM) is likely to be missed. If the 2-hour PG is >200 mg/dL in the early weeks of pregnancy, she may be a pre-GDM and glycated hemoglobin (HbA1c) of more than 6 is confirmatory. A pregnant woman found to have normal glucose tolerance (NGT), in the first trimester, should be tested for GDM again around 24th–28th week and finally around 32nd–34th week.

MANAGEMENT OF GDM

A team approach is ideal for managing GDM. The team would usually comprise an obstetrician, diabetes physician, a diabetes educator, dietitian, midwife and pediatrician.

Patient Education

The compliance with the treatment plan depends on the patient's understanding of:
- The implications of GDM for her baby and herself
- The dietary and exercise recommendations
- Self-monitoring of blood glucose
- Self-administration of insulin and adjustment of insulin doses
- Identification and treatment of hypoglycemia (patient and family members)
- Incorporate safe physical activity (walking at usual pace/arm exercise)
- Development of techniques to reduce stress and cope with the denial. Care should be taken to minimize the anxiety of the women.

Treatment

Target Blood Glucose Levels

In normal pregnancy, the mean plasma glucose (MPG) + 1 SD value for fasting is 89 mg/dL, and 2-hour is 122 mg/dL, hence maintenance of MPG level is approximately 105–110 mg/dL is desirable for a good fetal outcome. This is possible if FPG and 2-hour post prandial peaks are approximately 90 mg/dL and approximately 120 mg/dL, respectively.

Medical Nutrition Therapy

General principles: All women with GDM should receive nutritional counseling. The meal pattern should provide adequate calories and nutrients to meet the needs of pregnancy. The meal plan aims to provide sufficient calories to sustain adequate nutrition for the mother and fetus and to avoid excess weight gain and postprandial hyperglycemia. Approximately 30–40 kcal/kg ideal body weight or an increment of 300 kcal/day above the basal requirement is needed in 2nd and 3rd trimesters.

Calorie counting: This implies splitting the usual breakfast into two equal halves and consuming the portions with a 2-hour gap in between. By this the undue peak in plasma glucose levels after ingestion of the total quantity of breakfast at one time is avoided. More than 90% of GDM can be managed by medical nutrition therapy [MNT, Observation from the Diabetes in Pregnancy Awareness and Prevention (DIPAP) Project, supported by the Government of Tamil Nadu and World Diabetes Foundation (WDF)].

Initiating Insulin Therapy

Once diagnosis is made, MNT is advised initially for 2 weeks. If MNT fails to achieve control, i.e. FPG approximately 90 mg/dL and postmeal glucose approximately 120 mg/dL, insulin may be initiated (Flowchart 1).

MONITORING GLYCEMIC CONTROL

The success of the treatment for a woman with GDM depends on the glycemic control maintained with meal plan or pharmacological intervention. Studies suggest 1, 1½ and 2 hour postmeal for monitoring glycemic control. 2-hour postmeal monitoring is preferred as the diagnosis of GDM is also based on 2-hour plasma glucose. It is easier to remember this timing, as the time for diagnosis and also for monitoring is the same, i.e. 2 hours.

They should be advised to perform self-monitoring of blood glucose (SMBG) on a daily basis, failing which, at least weekly monitoring should be encouraged. If self-monitoring is not possible, laboratory venous plasma glucose has to be estimated for adjusting the dose of insulin.

Oral Antidiabetic Drugs

Insulin Secretagogue (Glibenclamide)

A randomized unblinded clinical trial compared the use of insulin and glyburide in women with GDM who were not able to meet glycemic goals on meal plan. Treatment with either agent resulted in similar perinatal outcomes. All these patients were beyond the first trimester of pregnancy at the initiation of therapy and publications on other drugs belonging to this group are dismal.

Metformin

A randomized controlled study found that in women with GDM, metformin (alone or with supplemental insulin) was not associated with increased perinatal complications as compared with insulin. Metformin has been found

Flowchart 1: Management of gestational diabetes mellitus.

A. Preferable to start with premix insulin 30/70 of any brand*

↓

Starting dose: 4 units before breakfast

↓

Every 4th day increase 2 units till 10 units

↓

If FPG remains >90 mg/dL advised 6 units before breakfast and 4 units before dinner

↓

Review with blood sugar test adjust dose further

↓

Total insulin dose per day can be divided as 2/3 in the morning and 1/3 in the evening

↓

Initially if postbreakfast plasma glucose is high start premix 50/50

↓

B. If GDM is diagnosed in the third trimester, MNT is advised for a week insulin is initiated if MNT fails

↓

C. If 2-hour PG >200 mg/dL at diagnosis, a starting dose of 8 units of premixed insulin could be administered straightaway before breakfast and the dose has to be titrated on follow-up. Along with insulin therapy, MNT is also advised

Note:
1. Usually women with gestational diabetes do not require >20 units of insulin per day for glycemic control, in comparison to type 1 and type 2 pregnant women whose daily requirement of insulin may be high.
2. Pregestational diabetic women during pregnancy may require high dose of insulin. A few may require multiple-daily injections (MDIs), usually given as short-acting insulin before breakfast and lunch and intermediate-acting insulin or premix before dinner.
3. Insulin dose is always individualized and has to be adjusted on follow-up.
4. If insulin requirement drops, placental insufficiency or fetal jeopardy has to be suspected (may also be due to increased utilization of maternal glucose by the supercharged beta cell mass of the macrosomic fetus—"*fetal handling of maternal glucose*").

to be useful in women with polycystic ovarian disease (PCOD) who failed to conceive. Continuing this drug after conception is still a controversy, but there are a few studies favoring continuation of metformin throughout pregnancy in these women. More studies are required before routinely recommending oral antidiabetic drugs during pregnancy.

Measuring Other Parameters

Maternal

Glycated hemoglobin level will be helpful to differentiate between a pregestational diabetic and GDM. If the HbA1c level is more than 6%, she is likely to be a pre-GDM. HbA1c is useful in monitoring the glucose control during pregnancy, but not for the day-to-day management. HbA1c level may serve as a prognostic value.

The blood pressure has to be monitored during every visit. If blood pressure is found to be more than 130/80, advise alpha-methyldopa 125 mg and dose to be adjusted on follow-up. Examination of the fundus and estimation of microalbuminuria, every trimester is recommended particularly in women with pregestational diabetes.

Fetal

Fetal Surveillance

Ultrasound fetal measurement: Ultrasound monitoring is recommended every trimester. A fetal echo is a must at 24 week, especially in prediabetics to rule out cardiac defects. In addition, documenting fetal biophysical profile in the late trimester is advisable. Doppler umbilical blood flow measurement or cardiotocograph (CTG) may be performed around 36 weeks of gestation in GDM with other pregnancy complications such as preeclampsia, hypertension, antepartum hemorrhage and intrauterine growth retardation.

Timing of Delivery

There is a possibility that the diagnosis of GDM may lead to increased obstetric intervention, including induction of labor and cesarean section. Delivery before full-term is not indicated unless there is evidence of macrosomia, polyhydramnios, poor metabolic control or other obstetric indications (e.g. preeclampsia or intrauterine growth retardation).

Delivery: During labor, it is essential to maintain good glycemic control (Table 2) while avoiding hypoglycemia. Lower insulin requirements are common during labor (often no insulin is necessary). Maternal blood glucose level should be monitored after delivery, 24 hours postpartum and if found to

Table 2: Plasma glucose and insulin IV fluid.

Plasma glucose At time of onset of labor	*Insulin/IV Fluids*
<70 mg/dL	5% GNS: 100 mL/hour
90–120 mg/dL	NS: 100 mL/hour
120–140 mg/dL	NS: 100 mL/hour plus *4 units of regular insulin added with IV fluid*
140–180 mg/dL	NS: 100 mL/hour plus *6 units of regular insulin added with IV fluid*
>180 mg/dL	NS: 100 mL/hour plus *8 units of regular insulin added with IV fluid*

Drip rate: 16–20 drops per minute. Maternal capillary blood glucose to be checked by glucometer every 1 hour and drip rate adjusted.

be high, checked again on follow-up. A neonatologist's presence at the time of delivery is ideal, more so if significant neonatal morbidity is suspected.

Neonatal Management

The neonates of mothers with GDM are also at risk of all complications similar to the infants born to mothers with overt diabetes, particularly those infants born macrosomic. In the Indian population, the normal birth weight of new born babies is between 2.5–3.5 kg. Neonates should be monitored closely after delivery for respiratory distress. Capillary blood glucose (cut-off of 44 mg/dL, i.e. 2.6 mmol) should be monitored at 1, 2 and 4 hours after birth and then again before feeding. Early breast feeding is actively encouraged.

FOLLOW-UP OF GDM

Gestational diabetes mellitus may be viewed as:
- An unidentified preexisting disease, or
- The unmasking of a compensated metabolic abnormality by the added stress of pregnancy, or
- A direct consequence of the altered maternal metabolism stemming from the changing hormonal milieu.

Gestational diabetic women require follow up. An OGTT with 75 g oral glucose, using WHO criteria for the nonpregnant population should be performed at 6–8 weeks postpartum. If found normal, GTT is repeated after 6 months and every year to determine whether the glucose tolerance has returned to normal or progressed. A considerable proportion of gestational diabetic women may continue to have glucose intolerance.

It is important that women with GDM be counseled with regard to their increased risk of developing permanent diabetes. Indian women with GDM have a high risk of developing diabetes (especially type 2 DM), and metabolic syndrome at a comparatively young age. They should be made aware of the symptoms of hyperglycemia and advice should be given about the importance of healthy eating and exercise patterns. Contraceptive advice and counseling regarding planning future pregnancies should be given. To avoid occurrence of neural tube defect in an unplanned pregnancy, 0.4 mg dose of folic acid is recommended on a daily basis by Center for Diabetes Control for all women of child-bearing age. The daily requirement of vitamin B12 during pregnancy is 2.6 μg which may not be available in a vegan diet. Hence, multivitamin tablets containing the required amount of B12 in addition to other vitamins may be recommended. Medical review by a family physician before conception, i.e. a preconception OGTT should be considered.

Preventive measures against type 2 DM should start during intrauterine period and continue throughout life from early childhood. In conclusion, a short-term intensive care gives a long-term pay off in the primary prevention of obesity, IGT and diabetes in the offspring, as *preventive medicine starts before birth.* The maternal health and fetal outcome depends upon the care by the committed team of diabetologists, obstetricians and neonatologists.

FURTHER READING

1. Dornhorst A, Rossi M. Risk and Prevention of Type 2 Diabetes in women with Gestational Diabetes. Diabetes Care. 1998;21(Suppl 2):B43-9.
2. Buchanan TA, Xiang A, Kjos SL, et al. "What is gestational diabetes?" Diabetes Care. 2007;30(2):S105-111.
3. Seshiah V, Balaji V, Balaji MS. Scope for prevention of diabetes–focus intrauterine milieu interieur. JAPI. 2008; 56:109-13.
4. Seshiah V, Balaji V, Balaji MS, et al. Pregnancy and Diabetes Scenario around the World: India. Int J Gynaecol Obstet. 2009;104(Suppl 1):S35-8.
5. Seshiah V, Balaji V, Balaji MS, et al. Prevalence of GDM in South India (Tamil Nadu)—A Community based study. JAPI. 2008;56:329-33.

Chapter 14

Neonatal Resuscitation: A Skill Every Obstetrician Should Know

Leena Das

INTRODUCTION

Mother and child are intimately related. In this busy schedule, obstetricians are the first person to receive a baby during delivery. So, all should be trained in the art of neonatal resuscitation. For each baby at least two persons are required if resuscitation is required. The first few minutes of extrauterine life is very vital for a baby. In intrauterine life baby was getting all its nutrient and oxygen from mother through placenta and was also in very warm environment. Suddenly everything is cut off and baby has to live in its own. About 90% babies cry on their own. About 9% require some assistance in the form of initial step, bag and mask ventilation, chest compression, only 1% requires extensive resuscitation-intubation and medication.

In newborn resuscitation, we have to look at *temperature, airway, breathing and circulation*. Newborns loose temperature rapidly by four ways: (1) conduction, (2) convection, (3) radiation, and (4) evaporation. For maintaining temperature, we have to keep the delivery room between 25° and 28°C, dry the baby immediately, wrap the baby or keep the baby in warmer/skin-to-skin contact.

ROUTINE CARE

About 90% of all babies start their respiratory effort immediately after birth. We have to only dry the baby, swipe the mouth and nose, cut the umbilical cord. Put the baby in mothers' abdomen immediately if the mother had normal delivery so that baby can take breastfeeding and maintain temperature by skin-to-skin contact. This also helps the mother in expulsion of placenta and reducing intrapartum hemorrhage.

If baby not cried immediately we have to do *"initial steps"*. We have to take the baby to the warmer. Put a 1 inch shoulder roll so that airway is patent.

Then clean the mouth and then the nose. Then dry the baby, if still not cried we have to give tactile stimulation twice in the sole or rub the back twice. Up to this step, we should do it in 30 seconds.

If still the baby is not taking respiration, we have to give positive pressure ventilation by bag and mask for 30 seconds. First 1 minute is the *"Golden minute"* of neonatal resuscitation.

Meconium-stained Vigorous Baby

In a baby born with *meconium-stained fluid,* who is *vigorous* [having a normal respiratory effort, good muscle tone, and a heart rate (HR) greater than 100 beats per minute (bpm)] may not need initial steps and can be observed with the mother.

Meconium-stained Nonvigorous Baby

In a depressed nonvigorous baby born with meconium-stained liquor, direct suctioning of the trachea soon after delivery is performed before any respiration has occurred. Follow these steps with other actions as discussed in initial steps of resuscitation. When these steps are followed appropriately, the risk of developing serious respiratory disorder may be considerably decreased.

Clearing Airway in a Nonvigorous Baby: The Following Steps need to be Followed

Clear the mouth using 12F or 14F suction catheter after inserting a laryngoscope to visualize the glottis. After the endotracheal tube has been inserted in trachea; attach it to a suction source. (You may need a special aspirator for this. Apply suction when the tube is in the trachea and slowly withdraw the tube continuing to apply pressure. This has to be done slowly over 3–5 seconds.

If the baby is breathing normally, check for HR. If HR is more than 100 beats/minute, see for color. If color is blue give free flow oxygen. Free flow oxygen can be given to a spontaneously breathing baby by using one of the following delivering methods:

- Oxygen mask
- Flow inflating bag and mask
- Oxygen tubing held close to the baby's nose and mouth with cupped hand
- T-piece resuscitator.

However, if ventilation is adequate in free flow oxygen but the baby still remains cyanotic, than a diagnosis of congenital cyanotic heart disease or persistent pulmonary hypertension of the newborn should be strongly considered.

If after initial steps the breathing has not started, we have to start *bag and mask ventilation* (Fig. 12.1).

Indication of positive pressure ventilation (PPV)—if HR less than 100 bpm or ineffective respirations. Initial pressure is 20–25 cm H_2O.

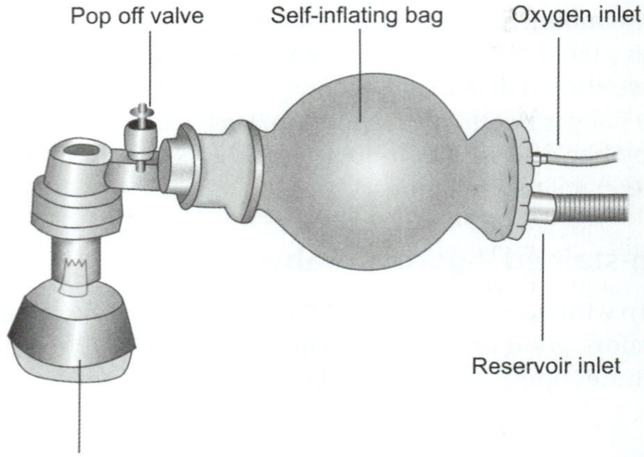

Fig. 12.1: Equipment required for bag-valve-mask ventilation.

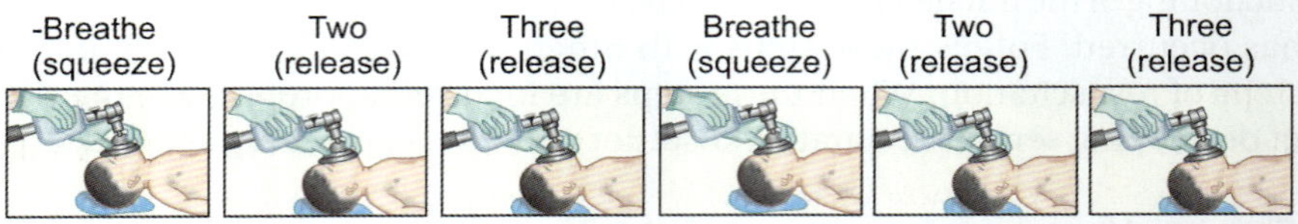

Fig. 12.2: Basic airway management—technique of bag-mask ventilation.

The *self-inflating bag* is presently the most commonly used ventilation device. The bag remains inflated following compression due to elastic recoil and does not need a compressed gas source to keep it inflated. It has a pressure limiting valve (pop off valve) regulated to limit inflation pressure to around 35–40 cm H_2O. The bag can be used with/without an attached manometer and/or oxygen reservoir. When squeezed, a self-inflating bag delivers a breath.

Appropriate Sized Face Masks

Masks come in a variety of shapes, sizes, and materials. An appropriate face mask must seal around the mouth and nose but not cover the eyes or overlap the chin. It can be difficult to establish and maintain a good seal between the mask and the infant's face and so it cannot be assumed that just because the mask is on the face, there is a good seal. Masks with a cushioned rim and round shape are preferable.

Providing Ventilation (Fig. 12.2)

- Squeeze the bag between thumb and two fingers using the dominant hand.
- Deliver a rate of 40–60 breaths per minute—call loudly "squeeze, two, three". Deliver a breath when you call squeeze and allow the bag to
- Use of shoulder roll to open the airway
- Applying face mask.

REMEDIAL STEPS

In case of *inadequate chest rise* look for
- Inadequate seal: Mask adjusted to ensure airtight seal
- Inappropriate position: Reposition the head in sniffing position
- Blocked airway: Suction the airway Open baby's mouth and ventilate
- Inadequate pressure: Increase pressure by squeeze the bag with more pressure till a chest rise is visible
- If no improvement with above steps, consider endotracheal intubation.

If PPV is prolonged over 2 minutes place an orogastric tube to prevent distention of stomach with air which may interfere with ventilation.

Contraindication of Bag and Mask Ventilation

- Diaphragmatic hernia
- Before suctioning of meconium stained nonvigorous baby.

OBSERVATIONAL CARE

If the baby has HR more than 100 beats/minute and have spontaneous respiration baby can be kept on observational care with mother, but vitals should be regularly monitored every half an hour.

Chest Compression

After 30 second of bag and mask ventilation if HR is less than 60 beats/minute consider chest compression along with bag and mask ventilation
- HR <60 bpm in spite of 30 seconds of effective PPV. Oxygen should be increased to 100%
- 2-thumb technique is still recommended. Once airway secured, switch to head of bed
- Electronic cardiac monitor preferred for assessment of HR
- Continue chest compressions for 60 seconds before rechecking.

Chest compression squeezes the heart between thoracic vertebra and sternum like an artificial pump. The depth of compression of sternum should be approximately one-third the anterior-posterior diameter of the chest.

Points to Note (Figs. 12.3A to C)

- Only two fingers tips should rest on the sternum
- Either the second hand or a hard surface should support the back
- Pressure is to be applied vertically.

The coordination of bag and mask and chest compression has to be done (Fig. 12.4).

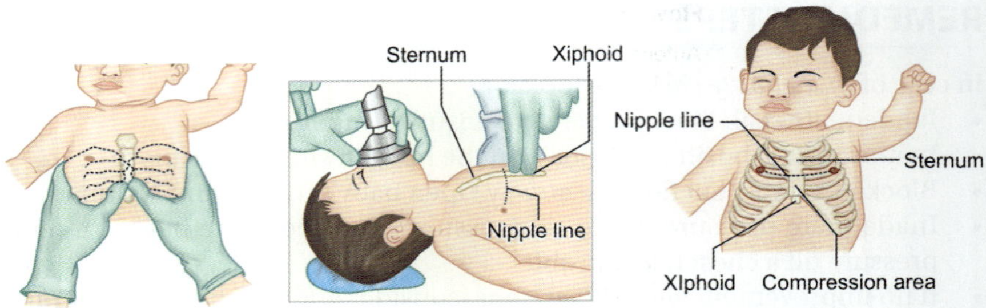

Figs. 12.3A to C: (A) Thumb technique; (B) Two finger technique; (C) Site for chest compression.

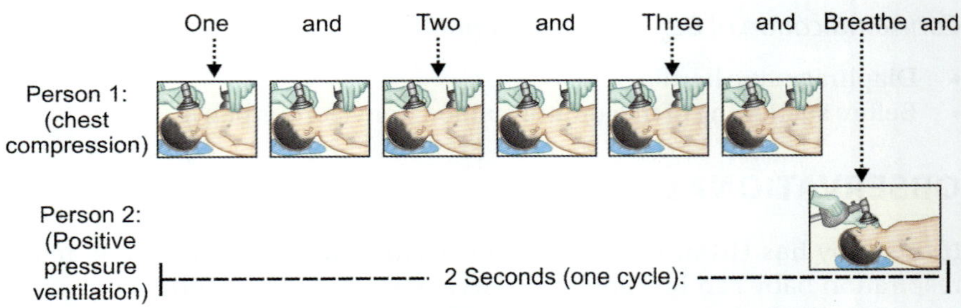

Fig. 12.4: Coordination of bag and mask and chest compression.

When to Discontinue Chest Compressions?

The HR should be above 60 bpm to stop chest compressions but the PPV is continued. After stopping the chest compression effective ventilation is delivered at 40–60 breaths/minute. Then ventilation is gradually stopped after HR goes above 100 bpm and the baby begins to breathe spontaneously. The baby is then shifted to neonatal intensive care unit (NICU)/ special care newborn units (SCNU) for post-resuscitation care.

If the baby is breathing, but has persistent respiratory distress (difficult breathing), attach a pulse oximeter (if available) to consider need for supplemental oxygen. If the baby is preterm, consider administering continuous positive airway pressure (CPAP) by face mask (if facilities available). If pulse oximeter and/or CPAP are not available, initiate supplemental oxygen and shift baby to NICU.

Acceptable Preductal SpO_2

- 2 min: 60%
- 3 min: 70%
- 4 min: 80%
- 5 min: 85%
- 10 min: 90%.

Flowchart 12.1: Neonatal resuscitation

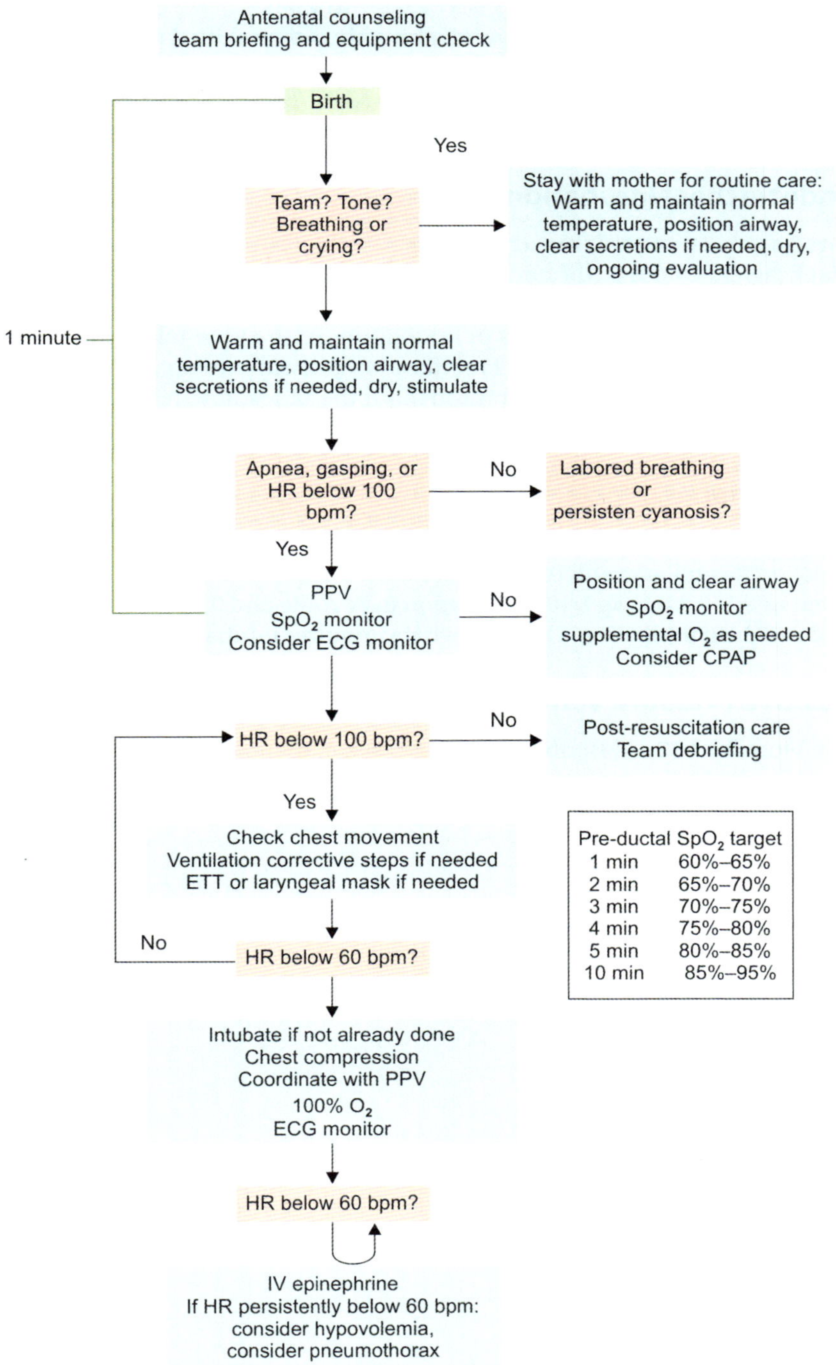

(ETT; endotracheal tube; HR, heart rate; ECG: electrocardiogram; PPV: positive pressure ventilation; CPAP: continuous positive airway pressure)

Post-resuscitation Care

- Preterm infants with labored breathing should be shifted to NICU/SCNU
- Newborns requiring PPV for more than 1 minute or needing intubation, or chest compressions should be shifted to NICU/SCNU for post-resuscitation care.

Endotracheal Intubation

Intubation is considered if prolonged ventilation is required and in diaphragmatic hernia. The endotracheal intubation will have to be completed quickly, preferably within approximately 30 seconds. The baby is not being ventilated during the attempts of intubation, so the time taken to intubate should be as short as possible. Free-flow oxygen with tubing at a flow rate of 5–6 L/min should be delivered throughout the procedure. It has to be done by a person who is expert.

Medication

Only normal saline and adrenaline is required. Nornal saline 10 mL/kg has to be given if capillary refill time is more than 3 second in bolus. Adrenaline is given as 0.1–0.3 mL/kg 1:10,000 dilution in IV route and 0.3–1 mL/kg through endotracheal intubation. Only 1% of baby requires intubation or medication.

Positive Pressure Ventilation

The Flowchart 12.1 describes neonatal resuscitation according to American Academy of Pediatrics.